Healthy Users

Healthy Users

THE GOVERNANCE OF WELL-BEING
ON SOCIAL MEDIA

Niall Docherty

UNIVERSITY OF CALIFORNIA PRESS

University of California Press
Oakland, California

Library of Congress Cataloging-in-Publication Data

Names: Docherty, Niall (Niall John), author.
Title: Healthy users : the governance of well-being on social media /
    Niall Docherty.
Description: Oakland, California : University of California Press,
    [2025] | Includes bibliographical references and index.
Identifiers: LCCN 2024059235 (print) | LCCN 2024059236 (ebook) |
    ISBN 9780520390621 (cloth) | ISBN 9780520390638 (paperback) |
    ISBN 9780520390645 (ebook)
Subjects: LCSH: Social media addiction—Prevention. | Well-being. |
    Internet users—Psychology. | Information technology—Social
    aspects.
Classification: LCC RC569.5.I54 D825 2025 (print) | LCC RC569.5.I54
    (ebook) | DDC 616.85/84—dc23/eng/20250122
LC record available at https://lccn.loc.gov/2024059235
LC ebook record available at https://lccn.loc.gov/2024059236

GPSR Authorized Representative: Easy Access System Europe,
Mustamäe tee 50, 10621 Tallinn, Estonia, gpsr.requests@easproject.
com

34   33   32   31   30   29   28   27   26   25
10   9   8   7   6   5   4   3   2   1

For Sophie

Contents

Acknowledgments

To begin, I'd like to say thank you to my teachers at Goldsmiths, University of London, who first gave me the confidence to explore my ideas during my undergraduate and postgraduate studies, in particular James Martin and Julia Ng, who mentored me during my early research projects, and Sanjay Seth, who initially planted the seed of a PhD in my mind.

The work of my PhD formed the theoretical basis for this book. Thanks go to my supervisors Jen Birks and Andrew Goffey at the Centre for Critical Theory, University of Nottingham, who helped guide me through the demands of the PhD with humor and dedication. My meetings with you furnished me with the (hard-learnt) skills to respond to criticism in a positive way, while also offering space to talk through challenging intellectual ideas with freedom. My thanks also go to Colin Wright and Helen Kennedy, who acted as internal and external examiners for my viva, respectively. This took place online in the strange early stages of the first UK lockdown. I enjoyed their virtual grilling as a welcome change of pace from the other online quizzes that populated my life back then.

I was lucky to be part of a great cohort of fellow PhD students at the University of Nottingham, and the groundwork for this book benefited from our lively discussions, regular WIPs, and the odd game of pétanque. Robert Stenson, Ivan Marković, Bettina Bódi, Niki Cheong, Louis Cotgrove, and Abi Rhodes in particular offered great companionship. Special mentions go to my good friends Joaquín Montalva Armanet and Magdalena Krysztoforska, whose teachings on Derrida and nonstandard epistemology continue to enrich my life today. Finally, to the man himself David Young—I thank you for your conversation and friendship.

My time at the Social Media Collective, Microsoft Research New England, was formative and offered a safe harbor to plan the research for this book in the years following my PhD. I thank Nancy Baym, Mary Gray, Tarleton Gillespie, and danah boyd for our weekly meetings and one-on-one-chats, where healthy use was often up for debate, as well as to Elizabeth Fetterolf, Rachel Bergmann, and Karina Rider for their solidarity and bants. Anna Gibson and Rida Qadri became great friends during my time in the US, and I am grateful for their guidance while I learned to walk the mean leafy streets of Cambridge, Massachusetts, while in the US. Further acknowledgments go to the lovely people I met through Microsoft Research, Dylan Mulvin, T. L. Taylor (who gave important feedback on the introduction of this book), Charlton McIlwain, Angèle Christin, Tawanna Dillahunt, Emily Tseng, Benjamin Ale Ebrahim, and Kate Sim. Finally, a special mention for Asia Biega, who taught me how to collaborate across disciplines, and for the rest of the members of the Responsible Computing Group at Max Planck, where I was a visiting fellow. This book would not have been possible without the input of all these colleagues.

I am grateful for the opportunity to have presented in-progress sections of this book at the invitation of various institutions. Particular thanks to the organizers and attendees of the Harvard Symposium on Social Media and Well-Being, the Oslo Digitox Seminar, and the AHRC Pause for Thought workshop (hosted by Thomas Sutherland and Scott Wark). At the University of Sheffield, thanks go to my friends and colleagues Jo Bates, Kate Miltner, and Susan Oman, who all offered valuable feedback on early drafts. Also my thanks to Rasmus Birk, who was a generous reader on the sections on idioms of distress. Likewise thank you to all members of the University of Sheffield Information School, the Digital Society Research Group, and the Digital Society Network at the University of Sheffield for providing a rich work environment for me to learn and write within. To all my students, thank you for providing the chance to talk through interesting ideas on a daily basis. And to all the professional service, estates, and facilities staff, thank you for making all these things possible.

At the University of California Press, my thanks go to Michelle Lipinski, who first approached me about a book project and who has always been generous with her time and support, and to Jyoti Arvey, who helped guide the manuscript to publication.

The research that has gone into this book is one thing, but it is the life and perspectives of everyone around me that I use as the inspiration for my work. On this, I reserve the most important thanks to my friends and family. Especially to my wife Sophie and our daughter Ruby—I would do anything for you both, but it just so happens that a small part of my contribution to our lives is to write for a living.

Introduction

Social Media Well-Being, Habit, Power

Good digital habits are critical to establishing and maintaining digital wellness.

META

These pre-existing forms of continuity, all these syntheses that are accepted without question, must remain in suspense. They must not be rejected definitively, of course, but the tranquillity with which they are accepted must be disturbed.

MICHEL FOUCAULT

At some point in your life, your habits have probably been a topic of conversation. Maybe you've been irritating someone, maybe that someone is trying to help. A parent, a teacher, a friend says: *You know you do this, right?* Brought to your attention, your habits can be changed. Softly or harshly, little tips for personal improvement are offered. *If you only did this, you could. If you stopped doing that, you would.* Habits are imagined as cultivars, with many interested in the type of character they create. Communities, families, educators, the state, institutions, private companies—whatever you like, all have a stake in what John Dewey once called "the interpenetration of habits" in the growth and construction of personhood.[1] Habits are the

[1]

stuff of conduct and, as such, could always be otherwise. This fluidity is often interpreted as an opportunity to exert control. Those who have a grip on their habits signal a well-disciplined body and mind. The opposite is true for those who do not. In recent times, habits have become a site through which individuals have been encouraged to attend to their health and well-being. Stop smoking, reduce your alcohol intake, get good sleep, eat well, exercise regularly, socialize, join a club—steps toward a longer life and a happier existence. In very recent times, we can add controlling our interactions with technology to this list. In particular, our engagements with social media (the most nefarious of them all) are said to require conscious attention and active management, lest we succumb to its toxic pitfalls and psychological traps.

"Social Media Could Be as Harmful to Children as Smoking and Gambling"; "Social Media Is a Parasite"; "Social Media Is Toxic."[2] Familiar headlines. Others, just as common, offer tips for digital self-improvement: "How Healthy Are Your Social Media Habits? 8 Tips to Upgrade Your Digital Wellness"; "Here's How to Tame Your Bad Tech Habit"; "How to Cut Back on Screen Time and Wean off Social Media."[3] In these framings, social media is an unhealthy, problematic technology, its users—the autonomous individuals they are—being responsible for their (un)healthy engagements with it. Much as with other perceived social vices, these headlines seem to indicate that the health risks of social media are both well understood and morally dubious. In particular, uncontrolled, unconscious, and unmanaged personal social media use is frequently linked to adverse psychological outcomes, such as increased user anxiety, depression, and loneliness.[4] In the face of these risks, it is time for you, the user, to get a grip on your digital habits and take control of your well-being online. Offering a helping hand, social media platforms have released various tools that encourage users to manage their online activity for the sake of their own good. Such tools are marketed as supporting conscious engagement, increased social communication, and balanced screen time on platforms. Users are especially encouraged to manage their social media activity through practices of self-tracking, active use, and ever more granular personalization of their social network feeds. Despite the apparent psychological risks that accompany social media use, it would seem that, given these tools and a degree of self-awareness, there are no excuses for not living well on platforms today. All it takes is a little discipline.

Yet this is too easy an answer to a misapprehended problem—and one that unfairly burdens individuals with its solution. This book will argue that the contemporary focus on personal habit as the key site of well-being interventions on social media, rather than constituting a simple equation of self-control, in fact reveals much broader and much more complex relations of power. Specifically, I will show how current discourses and designs of disciplined social media well-being function as part of historical apparatuses of *governance*.[5] This term, taken from the writings of Foucault, does not simply describe the work of legislative political entities, but refers to the various discursive material constraints and openings that shape human thought and activity in environments such as social media. *Governan*ce describes the operations of strategic micropower—the styles, manners, habits, negations, and directives encouraged and employed by individuals and groups to *conduct the conduct* of individuals and groups. Foucault refers to governance as the "modes of action, more or less considered and calculated," that are "destined to act upon the possibilities of action of other people," as deployed in certain ways, in certain locations, for certain goals.[6] Such activity works to affect the conditions of human existence without necessarily determining them, operating as much through aspiration and the targeting of desires as through punitive measures or moralized prescriptions. In the case of social media well-being, consider the ways in which digital wellness is positively promised to users if they adopt habits of active use, and how they are deemed personally failing and morally culpable if such a state eludes them. Through the ideas, tools, and habits of healthy use, pathways to the digital good life are laid, and we are duly assured that the psychological risks of social media can be managed by ourselves, acting alone, through our own willful self-control.

Yet, while the sole responsibility of individuals, striving toward healthy use is not only something that supposedly benefits users. More importantly, such healthy activity also works in the concrete interests of platforms themselves. Simplistically, capitalist social media platforms like Facebook, Instagram, and X make their money by transforming user interactions into data, which they can then sell to interested third parties for a profit.[7] This has been understood before in terms of *datafication*, where such processes, for instance, construct demographic insights able to facilitate targeted advertisements and messaging online, while also being used to tailor the content delivered to users on their feeds.[8] By ensuring that these profitable streams of datafication remain open through continued user engagements, healthy active use contributes to the continued economic flourishing of social media companies in their capacity as *data platforms*.[9] This is the strategic function of the governance of well-being on social media. Healthy use is profitable. Healthy users are profitable. Because of this, how these practices and roles are constructed and habitualized, respectively, is of crucial significance to the study of social media well-being, as well as to the broader study of how social media channels and expresses power in particular directions, shaping human life through particular means and aiming toward particular ends.

In this book, I will examine the intricacies and implications of the governance of well-being on social media through a triple-tiered empirical analysis of one particular platform: Facebook. I will combine textual content analysis, platform-interface analysis, and qualitative data created through interviews with British Facebook users to explore how healthy use, and the production of healthy users, is discursively and materially constituted. I will relate these findings to other, similar social media to argue that commercialized platforms' visions and tools of user wellness should not be taken at face value. Instead, I will show how the focus on individual user habits as the key correlate of well-being online works to both maintain and publicly diminish platforms' datafied capitalist operations, while simultaneously positioning psychologized practices of *neuroliberal* behaviorism as the prime modality through which users should imagine and attend to their well-being online today.[10] This has worrying implications that I will explore in this introduction and scrutinize throughout the book.

As conceived by scholars working in the field of human geography, neuroliberalism examines how behavioral psychology has come to be incorporated in the logics and practices of governance in the present day. In particular, neuroliberalism explores "the increasing capacity of states, corporations, and non-governmental organisations to govern through a series of more-than-rational registers of human action (including habits, heuristics, emotions, affects, and social and environmental contexts), and to skillfully fuse behavioural power with liberal notions of freedom."[11] Studies of neuroliberal governance look at how the habits of human beings have become contested sites of administration in organizational settings, paying special attention to how the attempted cultivation of baseline normalities furthers the interests and ideations of political, cultural, and social institutions. Studying how habits of social media well-being are encouraged and enacted, then, is a way to link various scales of analysis beneath one conceptual rubric, demonstrating their normalizing intersections and contingent characters. In particular, and as the term implies, this involves reckoning with the historical development and continued dominance of globalized *neo*liberalism, within which social media has emerged as a hegemonic form of social organization in the present.

Neoliberalism denotes the prioritization of marketized human freedom in Western domains, and beyond, for at least the past forty years.[12] Many have productively linked its ideological parameters to the types of social media emerging from Silicon Valley during the mid- to late 2000s and since (including Facebook).[13] In particular, this often relates to the tendency for social media to exacerbate practices of competitive individualism, performative displays of self-interested sociality, and consumptive media logics.[14] These overlaps reveal the fecundity of neoliberalism as a "scheme of reason" in contemporary spheres of human life, insofar as it motivates a set of marketized policy directives as well as the edification of entrepreneurialism as the prime heuristic for interpreting human activity and sociality.[15]

My engagement with *neuro*liberalism can help contextualize and pinpoint the key psychological tactics through which the governance of well-being on social media responds to and mobilizes some of these tropes. In doing so, and inspired by the work of Peter Miller and Nikolas Rose, I will treat the discourses, designs, and habits of social media well-being as examples of the "mechanisms through which authorities have sought to shape, normalize and instrumentalize the conduct, thought, decisions and aspirations of others in order to achieve the objectives they consider desirable."[16] More precisely, the lens of neuroliberalism will allow this book to (1) highlight how users interacting with social media are encouraged to understand, relate to, and modify themselves as healthy subjects; (2) examine the psychological rhetorics of justification behind these encouragements; (3) track the techniques of habit materialized in platforms for users to enact; and (4) examine where these practices come from and the relations of power, styles of existence, and economic outcomes they produce.[17]

Specific methods of sociotechnical script analysis from science and technology studies (STS) will help reveal the discursive materiality of these relations.[18] Drawing on the work of Madeleine Akrich in particular, we will see how the normative ideas that surround social media well-being, as well as its actual practice, redistribute existing forces in certain directions at the expense of others, being equally expressed through the design of platforms and in the discourses that constitute them. The domain knowledge and empirical focus of digital well-being studies and digital detox and disconnection studies will add an important scholarly backdrop to some of the concerns of this book, yet I will also apply the politicized impetus of poststructural cultural studies to add a greater critical depth to their empirical objects of study.[19] Through this interdisciplinary combination, if such a term carries any real meaning, I hope to offer readers a fresh analytical distance from the overly moralized terms of the current social media well-being discussion, offering an opportunity to objectify, reflect upon, parry, and divert its felt pressures in new ways. I will not weigh in on this side or that of the debate, nor will I suggest practices that are good for users or those they should avoid. Instead, the type of self-help found in these pages—to borrow an unfortunate appellation—provides alternative theoretical and empirical postures that can potentially reconfigure social media well-being into more manageable, less ardent, less admonishing forms. Overall, I will argue that a broader focus on the historical relations of power within which current debates of social media well-being are conceived can give a clearer picture of its present-day significance and help better shape its critical interpretation in the future.

I will detail the methodological approach of this book in more depth toward the end of this introduction. First, though, I will outline how the problem of social media well-being is currently constructed in contemporary mediatized debates, laying out the psychologized stakes of the present issue. I will show how control of personal social media habits is overwhelmingly presented as the primary correlate of user well-being. I will demonstrate how this position is expressed by social media companies, media outlets, health practitioners, governmental voices, industrial research scientists, some academics, and other interested stakeholders. Adopt conscious social media practices, the story goes, and you will live the good life online. Let social media determine your actions, however, and you will face the negative consequences. In this narrative, passive social media habits, such as unconscious scrolling, are said to result in reduced well-being and other negative psychological outcomes. Conversely, active use of platforms, including increased communications with loved ones, is said to lead to enhanced well-being, as measured in terms of increased social connection and decreased loneliness. In this way, the problem of social media well-being is overwhelmingly conceived as a matter of individual responsibility, and individual responsibility alone.

You may expect the many vocal critics of social media to offer alternatives to this portrayal, especially those who critique the *dark patterns* of social media design, which are said to capture, exploit, and drain the attention of users for economic gain.[20] However, this introduction will reveal how even those seemingly opposed to the economic machinations of social media are similarly trapped within the individualistic binary of active/passive use trumpeted by platforms themselves. I will argue that this troubling parallel is responsive to a key characteristic of neuroliberal governance in the present day: responsibilization.[21] Here, *responsibilization* refers to making individuals responsible for managing health risks that were previously the concern of others, such as the extended family, communities, or the state.[22] Responsibilization, in other words, is what follows from the attempted dissolution of community bonds and public institutions wrought through neoliberal policies, practices, and logics.

Throughout this book, I will highlight how current discourses and designs of self-controlled well-being management on social media have been forged within this historico-political context, binding individual users to the apparatuses of governance produced therein. I will argue that aligning well-being on social media solely with personal activity on platforms produces significant ideological effects, while also limiting the empirical scope and saliency of the issue in general. In summary, I will argue that a strict focus on user activity as the key determining factor of well-being on social media excludes any consideration of how platforms are actively involved in the shaping of the activities they support for economic purposes, or the ways in which well-being is experienced differently by users according to their different subjectification in social contexts—for example, through markers of race, class, gender, and physical capacity, among others, as they interact with local conditions. By treating well-being on social media purely in terms of healthy habits, that is, we ignore any consideration of how the capitalist infrastructures of social media are involved in the activation of such habits—how they produce, govern, and profit off the styles of life they support—and we are made blind to the social determinants of health that impact users unevenly due to historical inequalities and inherited privilege, prior to their arrival on platforms in the first place.[23]

However, although interconnected and keenly felt, these current responsibilized configurations of healthy social media use are by no means set in stone. I will engage in a Foucauldian mode of critique that, in the words of Ben Golder, problematizes "the discourses and modes of being that have come to define our present (and our relations to our present)."[24] I do so not only to "explain the various historical processes that have led to the current conjuncture of why we are, behave, or think in a particular way, but rather, and more pertinently, to defamiliarize and destabilize that conjuncture, to explain how it was produced and, by doing so, open it to the possibility of its being otherwise."[25] As such, the purposely destabilizing empirical analyses that I present throughout this book will show how current conjunctures of social media well-being are, in fact, "held together more by contingencies than by necessities, more by the arbitrary than by the obvious."[26] By highlighting these contingencies, and providing a more accurate cartography of their parameters, I aim to reveal strategic pressure points for those seeking to alter the forms they may take in the future. I will argue that when we recognize that contemporary neuroliberal capitalist cultivars of healthy use are not as inevitable or natural as some interested voices insist, we can imagine different modes of use (or of escape) capable of managing the impact of social media on well-being in daily life. To paraphrase Foucault, this book is engaged in an effort to reveal that the governance of well-being on social media can be changed, fragile as it is, and fragile as all things, really, are.[27]

Well-Being

This book will treat contemporary appeals to social media well-being as a *localized* proposition, recognizing that what *well-being* means fluctuates over time and place. Even within the narrow parameters of an individual life, personal ideas and praxis of well-being will change, perhaps even from one day to the next. In more philosophical terms, this variance is to say that models of well-being mobilize assorted ontological, epistemological, and axiological elements.[28] First, well-being is an ontological prospect insofar as any proposed benefits of well-being, and the practices that accompany it, require imagined "beings" to benefit. Second, the endeavor to know, measure, and compare this being in relation to others is an epistemological task. And third, due to the inherent normative directions of living well, as opposed to living poorly, discourses of well-being involve axiological statements of value. Therefore, examinations and evaluations of well-being render definitions of what the human is and what modes of conduct they should value.[29] This holds whether such elements are explicitly acknowledged or not.

Models of well-being, moreover, by being historically constituted, necessarily arise in response to temporal environmental, technological, social, cultural, religious, spiritual, and political exigencies.[30] Because *well-being* cannot be considered a stable term, as
something that self-evidently stands in for the human good, this
book moves away from its nominal examination and more toward its
operationalization in different spheres. Rather than quibble over
what social media well-being *really* is, I want us to instead question
what work different concepts of social media well-being are doing
when invoked at different times, by different people, institutions,
and groups. Inspired by the Foucault quote at the beginning of this
chapter, this book will hold the various conjoined ideas and techniques of social media well-being in analytical stasis, in order to better disassemble their qualities and examine their effects. Why this
version of social media well-being? Why now? Where? For whom?
And with what effects?

To establish what specific figure of the human is at stake in popular discourses of social media well-being, how such humans are supposed to be known, and what style of existence they are meant to
value, the next section will briefly examine the psychological literature on the subject that most clearly articulates this. In what follows,
we will be able to discern some of the dominant beliefs, or *sociotechnical imaginaries*, that currently structure the social media well-being
debate.[31] Sheila Jasanoff defines sociotechnical imaginaries as "collectively held, institutionally stabilized, and publicly performed visions of desirable futures, animated by shared understandings of
forms of social life and social order, attainable through, and supportive of advances in science and technology."[32] These imaginaries express not only collective hopes, but also fears. In the case of social
media well-being, many of these hopes and fears play out in
what Nikolas Rose calls the psy-disciplines, in particular the fields
of human-computer interaction (HCI) and social, computational,

cognitive, and behavioral psychology.[33] The findings from these myriad disciplines, whether proclaiming the virtues of social media connection or expounding its negative effects, are frequently taken up by media commentators, social media companies, regulators, critics, scholars, and, indeed, individual users as operative frames of reference in public conversations about healthy social media use.

You've probably bore witness to, or been involved in, some of these conversations. Perhaps a well-read friend or colleague has offered insights about the psychological impact of social media, positive or damaging, accompanied by recommendations of how to either cultivate or mitigate the effects. In what follows, I am not interested in either endorsing or debunking the findings upon which such recommendations are built. Instead, I will examine how they are mobilized in certain "games of truth" by various actors for various ends, and how such findings are used to validate and verify contemporary discourses and designs of healthy social media use.[34] Upon this basis, the following chapters will investigate how certain forms of knowledge work to justify communicative, technical, and moral well-being interventions in the lives of social media users.[35] With all this in mind, let us begin.

Active / Passive Use and the Psychological Controversies of Social Media

Several systematic and critical literature reviews, encompassing studies undertaken in roughly the first two decades of the twenty-first century, can offer some guidance on how social media well-being is currently constructed in the psy-disciplines.[36] In such studies, we frequently see different dimensions of well-being parsed out into distinct psychological categories, measured through various scales, and then variously correlated with the frequency, type, and intensity of use of particular platforms. Categories of user well-being measured on social media include self-esteem, life-satisfaction, social capital, positive and negative affect, happiness, self-acceptance, perceived autonomy, personal growth, and many more. These types of studies examine how these particular dimensions of well-being track onto particular forms of use of platforms. For example, as already mentioned, a common, and not uncontroversial, distinction is made between "active" and "passive" use.[37] These terms largely do what they say on the tin. *Active use* involves keen engagement with the diverse functions of social media platforms: communicating with loved ones, sharing photos, commenting on posts, liking, following, and so on. *Passive use*, on the other hand, denotes inactive engagement, such as lurking on other social media profiles with little or no interactions at all.

Some studies, including those undertaken by social media companies themselves, seem to show that active use of social media is correlated with various improvements in user well-being—increased scores of Subjective Well-Being (SWB), for example, which aims to capture measures of happiness, life satisfaction, and social capital. Such findings are frequently referenced by social media companies to indicate that higher levels of active use on their platforms equal higher levels of happiness and well-being in users, with the opposite being true for passive use. It is how you use social media that is said to matter here, nothing more, nothing less. Such findings are primarily explained by referencing the supposedly innate sociality of human users. The more social you are online, the more you are said to cultivate your biologically required social connections and related feelings of evolutionary species-belonging. The sweeping evolutionary ideas surrounding active/passive use will be fully explicated (and critiqued) in subsequent chapters, and it is important to note that this binary has been contested before.[38] Yet it remains that many of the present-day concerns over the impact of social media on user well-being are similarly developed in terms of the facilitation, disruption, type, and scale of active/passive human sociality afforded by platforms. A major framing of this issue is in terms of social comparison, whereby one processes information about others "in relation to the self."[39] In particular, the opportunity for increased (and potentially limitless) social comparison on social media has frequently been associated with negative psychological outcomes, such as increasing levels of envy in users or the depreciation of certain psychological classifications, such as body image, particularly in youth.[40] In more clinical domains, one meta-analysis of psychological studies of Facebook found that "upward social comparison" on the platform, whereby users compare themselves with others they see as having higher social status, can even be correlated with higher levels of depression.[41]

As well as these individual impacts, some suggest that social media proliferates hate as a prosocial phenomenon, facilitating mutually supporting communities to emerge around discriminatory beliefs.[42] Others examine how this damages the self-worth of targeted users, in particular the hate directed at nonheteronormative, nonwhite representations of femininity.[43] The impact of misinformation or conspiracy theories on the well-being of users has also been explored, with many linking the adversarial news environments of social media to increased stress, perhaps as a result of the extra cognitive load involved in deciphering the veracity of information sources.[44] Other stressors on social media include the perceived demand to be always connected and always available, which is said to aggravate the corresponding demands to fulfill idealized presentations of the self online.[45] That you only present the best version of yourself on social media is now an almost banal insight, but how these performances respond to hegemonic ideals of racialized and gendered body types, aspirational lifestyles, career success, and imagined popularity is a productive and valuable area of inquiry.[46] In particular, such presentations have been shown to serve a normative function through the metrification of likes, comments, and shares, with posts being stacked up against each other on semipublic feeds.[47] Life on social media, as such, becomes a competition, measured and ranked through the algorithmic ordering of user-generated content, creating environments where increased attention on posts is often felt as a personal success, and obscurity felt as a failure.[48]

In more medicalized spheres, various types of social media use, for various demographics of users, are regularly mapped onto categorizable dimensions of mental health.[49] Such studies may explore, for example, how social media use and communication correlate with greater or lesser degrees of rumination, anxiety, narcissism, depression, disordered eating, social phobia, and other affective and personality disorders.[50] Using similar explanatory frameworks regarding the social nature of human beings introduced above, some of these studies assume that social media provides users an enhanced opportunity to reflect upon their personal position in relation to others in a social network, often leading to negative, and sometimes unmanageable, feelings of inadequacy and diminished self-worth as a result.[51] The perils of "too much" social media run in parallel to the anxieties over "too much" screen time overall, especially for adolescents.[52] These fears run high, with some examining excessive screen time in relation to declining well-being and decreased concentration, and others, such as Jonathan Haidt, explicitly correlating rising mental health issues such as anxiety in teens with the increasing availability of the smartphone—especially in the US.[53] Others identify the negative physical effects of scrolling, swiping, and other haptic social media habits on the bodies, senses, and posture of users, including specific issues to do with eye strain and neck flexion from mobile scrolling, for example, or the negative impact of social media on sleep patterns.[54]

As we can see, the psychological issues of social media are myriad, variously linked to individual threats and population-scale crises in turn. However, this is not the full picture, and elsewhere we find studies that focus on the potentially beneficial aspects of social media for well-being. For instance, some argue that practices of social comparison on social media could conceivably work in a more positive manner, specifically by allowing users to situate themselves more accurately within their own social context, or by providing sources of social inspiration.[55] Others highlight the potential well-being benefits of developing parasocial relationships with public figures on social media, which can lead to interactive communities forming around them online.[56] The facilitation of peer support on social media has been shown to benefit different demographics of users with shared experiences—for example, for users undergoing cancer treatments.[57] Some argue that the simple ability to communicate with family and loved ones who do not live in close physical proximity can lead to many psychosocial benefits.[58] Recently, and in response, some scholars have even begun examining social media well-being in terms of its eudaimonic dimensions—understood as those practices that lead to positive flourishing and feelings of long-term fulfillment for individuals.[59]

As I have already indicated, I am not concerned with debating the reproducibility or validity of this research emerging from the psy-disciplines. I am also not planning to mete out advice upon the basis of these resources in response. Instead, I am interested in what assumptions these studies mobilize, how they produce certain epistemological prisms through which we are led to understand the impact of social media on the well-being of users at large, and how these understandings justify particular social media well-being discourses and designs as a result. With this in mind, it is important to note that problematic social media use is often viewed as part of a broader picture of mental health for the individuals examined, with social media exacerbating certain psychological symptoms as well as the proclivity to experience them, rather than simply causing them in isolation.

For example, some scholars working in the psy-disciplines take a situated approach in order to explain how diverse experiences of social media well-being reflect societal inequalities and historical forms of intersectional discrimination. These include works that explore how reported scores of social media well-being relate to experiences of racial discrimination, online and offline; how differences in geographic localities influence social media well-being, such as those extant between users residing in the Global South and those residing in the Global North; or the ways in which misogyny impacts the perceived and actual safety of social media platforms for gendered subjects.[60] Other scholars advocate socioeconomic status as a pertinent category in the measurement of social media well-being, with digital inequality examined as if it were, indeed, reflective of societal inequality writ large.[61]

To examine these issues is to treat social media well-being as a culturally and socially constrained set of holistic relations—comprising intersecting dimensions of race, class, disability, and sexuality, among others—interacting with material circumstances such as education, employment, and housing. Making these relations explicit is an important critical intervention, not to mention an empirically valuable step, as marginalization in any of these interconnected aspects of life can be productively linked to increased states of stress online. These increased states of stress, as public health scholars have shown, can be subsequently linked to an increased likelihood that epigenetically activated mental health issues will emerge in impacted populations.[62] Basically, living in environments hostile to certain ways of life takes its toll on the well-being of differently situated individuals in uneven ways, well before they even think about accessing social media from wherever they are located. Although these examples of situated psychological investigations are obviously in no way exhaustive, they serve to illustrate how social media well-being can—and, as this book argues, should—be used to discuss wider networks and operations of power beyond the personal use of platforms and, indeed, beyond the personal control of users themselves.

Toxic Platforms

Despite the existence of this more situationally attuned research, media outlets in the anglophone Global North, which is the broad analytical remit of this book, regularly come at the issue from a distinctly individualized perspective.[63] As opposed to viewing the issue holistically, popular imaginaries often emphasize how the stated toxicity of platforms chiefly interfere with discrete and internal psychological mechanisms. One exemplar is the *Wall Street Journal*'s 2021 "Facebook Files" series, which covered leaked internal documents from Meta that seemed to show the company was aware of the psychological harms that could be caused by using its services, focusing in particular on the dangers excessive social comparison could pose to teenage girls.[64] In this series, the metaphor of toxicity was frequently employed to describe how platforms could impact the psychological states of users, suggesting poisonous social media atmospheres where the basest aspects of human existence fester, spread, and demean all those who come into contact with them.[65] In these dramas of toxicity, misinformation, racism, misogyny, ableism, sexist imagery, and fake news largely circulate with impunity, with outrage about these issues, as well as their active endorsement, understood as notable drivers of the so-called attention economy.[66] Here, user clicks are said to form the foundation of economic value extraction for capitalist data platforms, leading some to question whether companies are at all interested in making their platforms safer spaces for users, considering the high value that online (attention-grabbing) fury produces within their business operations.[67] Platforms reply by referencing opposing business logics, claiming that they can only retain their user base if their platforms are welcoming places for communication (something later chapters will return to in more depth). Far from hiding their motivations, then, platforms argue that ensuring the well-being of their users makes solid business sense, insofar as healthy spaces, fostering healthy communication, create healthy profits.

Elected democratic governments have thus far struggled (or maybe refused) to legislate these issues comprehensively, largely focusing on enforcing companies to regulate legal but harmful content on their platforms, as evidenced by the UK's Online Safety Bill.[68] This can be understood in relation to the neoliberalized context within which governments and public health institutions in the Global North operate, where policies like the EU Digital Services Act demonstrate a reluctance to interfere in marketized spheres of online communication, beyond increased calls for transparency.[69] Following interviews with elected politicians in Norway, for example, Gunn Enli and Karin Fast revealed how user well-being is principally imagined by democratic legislators as an individual responsibility, rather than a potential site of policy intervention.[70] As already indicated, such ideas reflect historical discourses and practices of responsibilization, whereby welfare models of state intervention in public health have been dissolved in favor of the marketized provision of care.[71] With the state's obligation to care for its citizens diminished, responsibilized individuals are left to personally fulfill what Pat O'Malley describes as *the duty to be well* in their own lives, through their own means, and at their own risk.[72]

Such ideas of dutiful responsibility are implicit in advice given to parents about social media well-being by the UK's chief medical officer, for instance, which focuses on keeping family screen time "under control" in order to balance the potential costs and benefits of technologically mediated life.[73] Conveying a similar sentiment, a National Institutes of Health (NIH) News item from the US, tellingly titled "Healthy Social Media Habits: How You Use It Matters," argues that how users engage with social media is the major factor in its psychological impact.[74] To quote this piece, US citizens are advised by the NIH to use their time "wisely" on platforms by actively involving themselves in social communication and avoiding passive scrolling, while also being "careful" in who they choose to connect with and how. In such guidance, the dichotomy between active and passive use is in full effect. As a result of this, responsibility for social media well-being is placed squarely on the shoulders of individuals, despite the known factors that make life online more or less difficult for differently situated users in digital spheres.

All of this is to say that the way the issue of social media well-being has been taken up in public discourses presents a fairly blunt narrative. Personal feelings of well-being on social media, whether users have a positive relationship with social media or not, whether users are satisfied with their online lives, whether their usage leads to increased or lowered feelings of self-esteem, whether they are stressed out on platforms, happy, unhappy, comfortable, vexed, and so on, are all presented as the result of individual actions, decisions, and habits alone. Feeling anxious about your relationship status? Well, that's hardly surprising considering how much you lurk on your ex-partner's feed throughout the day. Maybe stop doing that. Getting depressed through comparing yourself with others? Stop passively staring, get active, and reach out to your social network. Struggling to sleep at night? Don't post before bed! Here, the various psychological issues that could be associated with certain types of social media use are said to be solved through making simple changes to individual habits. It's all a matter of self-control and cultivating the right style of use.

Platforms themselves are keen to share and spread the meritocratic doctrine of personal responsibility. Meta, for example, the parent company of Facebook, Instagram, and Whatsapp, dedicates a section of its online safety center to "Digital Wellness." Here, users are encouraged to "prioritize digital wellness" by cultivating active interactions on their feeds, practicing honesty in their posting, and following hashtags, friends, and pages that "inspire" them.[75] Other practical suggestions include balancing and managing screen time, chiefly by tracking, and maybe limiting, the time spent on platforms by using monitoring applications. Other commercial social media platforms like YouTube and TikTok provide similar tracking tools, wellness targets, and ways to encourage modes of conscious engagements for their users. Subsequent chapters will explore how social media companies validate their recommendations through appeals to knowledge constructed in the psy-disciplines, demonstrating how they are technically built into the design of user interfaces themselves. Moreover, I will examine the modes of responsibilization that these norms enforce, and critically examine how they ensure that the profitable avenues of user interaction remain open for platforms through the positive inculcation of engaged use. For now, I'd like you to hold on to the observation that the discourses and tools of social media well-being offered by companies all focus on users managing their own habits online, controlling their own screen time, and navigating the ostensible psychological risks of toxic platforms by their own wits and volition. In other words, I want you to hold in stasis the overarching claim made by Meta that opened this introduction: "Good digital habits are critical to establishing and maintaining digital wellness."

False Equivalence

This book argues that focusing solely on individual habits as the primary correlate of social media well-being ignores the wider social determinants of health that unevenly impact different users, in different ways, prior to their observable engagements with platforms. The social determinants of health framework, as described by the World Health Organization, suggests that "the conditions in which people are born, grow, live, work and age" are important factors in individually differentiated experiences of health.[76] These include relative terms of personal income, for instance, places of habitation, access to health care, access to education, scales of societal inequity, and environmental factors such as local levels of pollution.[77] It follows that access to social media necessarily occurs within these contextual settings. Social determinants of health are therefore salient factors in respective experiences of social media well-being for differently located and culturally situated demographics of users.

These relational views of health and well-being have been influential in the critical medical humanities, where they are often examined through complementary epigenetic concepts such as the *exposome*.[78] In the words of Rupa Marya and Raj Patel, the exposome refers to the "sum of lifetime exposure to nongenetic drivers of health and illness," encompassing the "chemical, social, psychological, ecological, historical, political, and biological elements" that trigger adverse health outcomes.[79] Marya and Patel focus on the way living in societies hostile to certain groups, peoples, and ways of life leads to increased exposure to psychological stressors. Resulting increases in stress have been shown to increase inflammation at a cellular level, which, in turn, has been associated with overstimulation within the immune system, itself leading to a higher risk of associated conditions and diseases as a result.[80] These medical approaches are complemented by the work of cultural theorists such as Sianne Ngai and Ann Cvetkovich, who examine the experience of human emotions, as well as mental health issues such as depression, as responses to the way power pressures individuals living in the same environments on radically different scales of intensity.[81]

Following this type of thinking, the possibility of living well online cannot solely depend on active use, conscious engagement, or controlled screen time. Rather, one can only live well on social media if the world within which social media exists allows you to do so—in the way that you would wish. This holistic stance is in stark contrast to the dominant reductive accounts of social media well-being outlined above. This book will understand this foreclosure as a form of *topical exclusion*, a term introduced by Foucauldian scholar Tuomo Tiisala to describe how power strategically produces interpretive vacuums within which interested parties can shape the narrative surrounding certain public controversies.[82] For Tiisala, "topical exclusion produces ignorance (about x) by directing attention (at y)."[83] Accordingly, strict correlations between social media well-being and controlled habits can be considered as part of newly uncovered "strategies of power," intentional or not, which "harness and produce ignorance" alongside, and often in conflict with, the generative functions of power/knowledge.[84] In this case, rather than interrogating the structural conditions that may be contributing to feelings of digital distress on social media for different users, all attention is instead focused on changing habits at the individual level, and the individual level alone. As a result, social media well-being loses its potency as a site of critical interpretation.

Responsibilized Parallels

It is hardly surprising that platforms correlate self-controlled use with social media well-being, lest attention be drawn to the possibility that their designs and business models could be partially culpable for the current psychologized malaise. However, when you look at how the issue is conceived by ostensible critics of social media, odd parallels can be observed. Chiefly, those who oppose the extractive economic functioning of social media are similarly stuck on individual habits as the primary safeguard against its perceived psychological ills. It seems that adopting good digital habits is unanimously presented as the primary path to positive well-being outcomes on social media, whether or not you actually endorse the operations of platforms themselves. As a consequence, no matter what stance you take, buying into the individualized terms of the current social media well-being debate results in the same damaging political effects highlighted above.

For example, the Center for Humane Technology, which was involved in the Netflix film *The Social Dilemma*, is a group of vocal critics who suggest that users "take control" of their social media habits for the sake of their own digital well-being.[85] With support available from a range of applications on the market, users are encouraged to manage the time they spend on platforms, set boundaries for their use, focus on the positive aspects of their interactions, and be compassionate in their communications. The only thing that sets these suggestions apart from platforms' own is how they are framed. Principally, critics highlight the difficulty of controlled use when individuals are up against toxic platform atmospheres and "addictive" designs. Critics reference the *dark patterns* of social media as pernicious tactics to keep users engaged online, which include alluring color schemes, push notifications, and the prioritization of appealing content on feeds. These features are said to be deeply embedded economic ploys, designed to keep users "hooked" on platforms for purposes of datafication.[86]

Nonetheless, despite the stated difficulty of the task, these recommendations assume that it is primarily the responsibility of users to first recognize the risks of social media and then get a grip on their interactions with it. The field of disconnection studies has examined how the widespread calls to take back control of our social media habits are variously expressed within media spheres—whether in a burgeoning self-help literature, as peddled within the influencer economy, or monetized through digital detox wellness retreats and corporate well-being strategies.[87] In particular, the call to resist the demands of social media, escape its extractive designs, and regain control has been understood against the backdrop of the ubiquitous digitality of the present day and its overriding neoliberalized tone. An individual's ability to handle these technological pressures successfully, for instance, has been studied as a quality that users can use to set themselves apart from a competitive social field, with several scholars locating the performative aspects of digital wellness within neoliberal regimes of individuated entrepreneurship of the self and self-interested social networking.[88]

Although popular critical voices situate suggested changes to user habit within a series of cascading interventions aimed to regulate the business practices of social media more broadly, it is the shared focus on controlling technological habits on both sides of the debate—and the political, social, and economic exigencies this topically excludes—that is at stake in this book.[89] Why is the call to adopt and control good digital habits so strong for these seemingly opposing camps? And how has individual activity come to be imagined as the principal solution to the majority of social media's psychological ills? As already indicated, this book argues that one of the chief reasons for this shared horizon is the prevailing hegemony of neoliberal responsibilization that frames digital wellness today, and in particular its focus on individual activity as the driving mechanism of change and source of accountability in public policy spheres today. Think here of the liberal democratic responses to the COVID-19 pandemic. In the UK as in other places, individual habits were targeted as a chief location of political regulation. Restrict your social contact, wash your hands, stop hugging. These individual changes were offered to citizens as a way to reduce the spread of COVID. In an approach founded on ideologies of nudge (to be disussed in later chapters), "choice architects" cajoled and shaped human behavior in the pandemic through the arrangement of social mores and contextual cues in environmental settings, perhaps instead of other more comprehensive and more effective policies.[90] Yet, beyond the debatable efficacy of nudge interventions, consider how responsibility for change is attributed within its purview. In the UK's response to COVID-19, consider the way the UK state withdrew from the management of the pandemic in a form of distanced paternalism—involved certainly, influential for sure, but somewhat removed from the measures' success or failure. Instead, individuals were made responsible for stopping the spread of the virus, with the moral imposition to make a difference in the course of the pandemic landing on their shoulders, however poorly prepared and however poorly provided for. In nudge, individual choices are both the cause and the solution to societal-scale problems.

Following Rose, such processes of responsibilized nudge, which encourage individuals along contingent behavioral routes, making them responsible for their actions and providing a psychological justification for doing so, ought to be considered as part of a "complex of apparatuses, practices, machinations, and assemblages within which the human being has been fabricated" throughout history.[91] That is, setting out habits that are supposedly good for people, and determining those that they should avoid, is to offer individuals a vision of who they are supposed to be. And through their successes and failures cultivating those habits, people are granted means to measure and understand themselves as successful or unsuccessful subjects. For Rose, this functions as an "intellectual technology," making "visible and intelligible certain features of persons, their conducts, and their relations to others" as desirable, and others as undesirable.[92] However, far from being only an internal normative relation, the discursive effects of these normative regimes make certain actions and thoughts more likely than others simply by their positioning above and against each other. This is the materiality of discourse. And because of these material effects—by making people up, by fashioning their activities, by constructing fields of possibility—psychological regimens of habit management and their enactment, such as contained in the delinations of self-controlled healthy use examined above, can be productively understood in terms of governance, the specificities of which I will turn to now.

Governance

Rather than simply describe the actions of governments, democratically elected or otherwise, or political policy decisions, and how those decisions are made and enforced, *governance*, following Foucault, instead refers to the *conduct of conduct*.[93] Governance, as Daniele Lorenzini writes, exists in the productive tension between three pivotal capacities: "to conduct someone, to (let oneself) be conducted, [and] to conduct oneself."[94] Accordingly, governance operates upon and through human freedom, not in spite of it.[95] One element of governance refers to the techniques and channels through which power incites people to operationalize their freedom to act for themselves, (as if) for their own ends. Foucault genealogically traces the emergence of these relations to the formation of the capitalist, marketized civil society in the West, whereby the problematics of liberal governance revolved around ensuring the independence of self-regulating domains (e.g., "civil society" or "the economy") and keeping the conditions of equal exchange between market actors in balance with the demands of the sovereign.[96] Subsequent scholars, as well as Foucault himself, have examined the historical development of these problematics into overlapping neoliberal governmentalities that question their own internal limits through "perpetual problematisation."[97] In doing so, these governmentalities have further constructed the conditions of financially marketized freedom for individual entrepreneurs to flourish, focusing on competition, self-improvement, risk, psychological aspiration, and efficient calculation as eminent values and practices for citizens to live by.[98]

Importantly, processes of governance regulate human freedom through the construction of subjects that are capable of being regulated. Foucault calls this process *subjectivation*, the "formation of a definite relationship of self to self."[99] Such self-relations, in turn, provide motivations and reasons for individuals to act in certain ways, making it more likely that those actions will occur in certain locations as a result. Interested actors—the state, institutions, corporations, social media companies, and so on—seek to shape these relations in order to effect certain ends. Governance is therefore not a top-down process, but rather is *enacted* in a lattice-like spread by agentic individuals. Productive power is charged with potential insofar as individuals are led to imagine themselves as beings with certain natural tendencies, capacities, and desires. Power is activated through governance in the extent to which subjects act upon these imagined tendencies or do not. With this in mind, as already hinted at above, this book engages with these ideas to examine the ways in which users of social media are prompted to conceive of themselves as healthy subjects, vulnerable to certain failings, and capable of self-improvement via certain habits as a result. In other words, we will explore how the promise of personal well-being is offered to social media users as a motivation to adopt practices of active (profitable) use on platforms.

Within analytics of governance, there is no sense that power is a closed circuit, always oppressive, or determined. Accordingly, we cannot locate a single origin of power in order to block or remove its force. Rather, power constitutes, makes, and molds. For Foucault, as such, "the exercise of power consists in guiding the possibility of conduct and putting in order the possible outcome."[100] Without recourse to locate the source, the wellspring of power, governmental analysis seeks to expose exactly *what* styles of life and subjects are being produced in different locales, how this occurs, who or what this works for to a greater or lesser extent, and who or what this restricts. In doing so, we may be able to identify weaknesses in the shape of governmental power and suggest strategic targets that are, more or less, more open to change than others.[101] Hence, there is no sense that humans can escape power, or become *more* free, only that they could, perhaps, feel and act upon their freedom in different forms.

Apparatuses of Power

The hope explored in this book, if you are looking for it, is that we may be able to locate new forms of well-being on social media that are more aligned with how different human individuals and groups would wish to be conducted and how they would wish to conduct themselves. We will explore if it is possible to identify new styles of social media well-being beyond its neuroliberal manifestations, or if there are other online habits that users can adopt that do not perpetuate the cycle of toxicity, responsibilization, and raw capitalist accumulation effected through daily social media use. Repeating a core assumption of this book, power can be imagined and shaped in other ways only if we have a clear picture of its current strategic functions. Because resistances are always immanent in the field of power relations under scrutiny, having a lucid view of its operations is of the utmost importance. Thinking ahead, the conclusion of this book will offer some "tactical pointers" as to what these resistances could conceptually and practically look like in the domain of social media well-being, specifically through the analytic of *counter-conduct* and alternative ethical subjectivations relating to *care of the self*.[102]

The view of productive power and freedom that undergirds this book stands in contrast to the ways in which the possibility of change is articulated in popular discourses and designs of self-controlled social media well-being, as found on both sides of the debate outlined above. A shared conceptualization of change is a crucial part of the reason why these opposite sides find themselves suggesting the same courses of action in response to the psychological risks of social media. Namely, the dichotomy between active and passive use and the demands to take back control of personal habits on platforms maps onto tired, yet still implicitly prevalent, frameworks of structure versus agency, which often stymies discussions of human technological relations today.[103] *Structure* here refers to the fixed technological possibility of platforms—their communicative functions, social affordances, and so on—while *agency* refers to the ability of users to wield these functions for their own ends.

In this binary, the potentially determining aspects of social media platforms reside in their inculcation of passive habits in users, which are imagined to override human freedom.[104] Power is said to flow in a vertical manner. Control is imagined to switch back and forth between the two poles of platforms and users respectively. Primarily, the ability of humans to recognize and advocate their own autonomy over technological tools is the key to whether they have power over them. As this manifests in the opposite yet parallel sides of the popular social media well-being debate, users either control the tools of social media or are controlled by them.[105] Such value-neutral views of technology as a tool place responsibility for proper healthy use of platforms in the hands of users.[106] This ends up repeating the tropes of responsibilization outlined above, topically excluding the social determinants of health in discussions of social media well-being, and perpetuating worldviews that imagine isolated users divorced from the social world around them. By employing alternative analytics of power in this book, and an alternative sociotechnical view of technology (that I will detail shortly), I hope to move beyond these conceptual limitations. In doing so, and building on a growing tradition of critical multidisciplinary social media research, I offer new ways to think through the bind of self-control that currently, and unfairly, burdens users to navigate the uneven pressures of social media well-being by themselves, alone, in the present day.

Accordingly, this book positions itself in contrast to *juridico-discursive* theories of power. [107] In brief, the juridico-discursive matrix, commonly operationalized in liberal democratic theory, legal frameworks, and in the debates surrounding social media self-control and structure versus agency, works upon the assumption that power chiefly exists as a negative externality, hierarchically centralized, that can be possessed and held over another. In contravention to this, Foucault argues that "power must be understood in the first instance as the multiplicity of force relations immanent in the sphere in which they operate and which constitute their own organisation."[108] Power, accordingly, is not something that can be studied in and of itself. It would be erroneous to question who *has* power or what they are doing with it. Instead, Foucault urges us to develop an *analytics of power* that seeks to assess the ways in which power shapes, transforms, strengthens, or reverses forms of human life and organization in distinct settings, at particular moments in time.[109]

"If power were never anything but repressive," Foucault questions, "if it never did anything but to say no, do you really think one would be brought to obey it? What makes power hold good, what makes it accepted, is simply the fact that it doesn't only weigh on us as a force that says no, but that it traverses and produces things, it induces pleasure, forms knowledge, produces discourse."[110] Upon this basis, power can be located in its effects, however general, wide, small, specific, or varied they may be. Power ought to be examined as the "the support which these force relations find in one another, thus forming a chain or a system, or on the contrary, the disjunctions and contradictions which isolate them from one another."[111] Foucauldian-inspired analytics are particularly attentive to the strategic function of power, not as a unilateral imposition, but as a response to particular events, crises, shifts in thinking, technological disturbances, and other temporal phenomena, such as the controversies over social media well-being in the present day.

Foucault encompasses these shifting relations through his nebulous (and infamous) concept of the *dispositif*, otherwise known as the *apparatus.*[112] Through the apparatus, an approach to problems or "urgent needs" appears that seeks to establish links, relations, and dependencies between a set of elements that would otherwise have been seen as heterogeneous.[113] "The apparatus," Foucault writes,

> is essentially of a *strategic* nature, which means assuming that it is a matter of a certain manipulation of relations of forces, either developing them in a particular direction, blocking them, stabilising them, utilising them, etc. The apparatus is thus always inscribed in a play of power, but it is also always linked to certain coordinates of knowledge which issue from it but, to an equal degree, condition it. This is what an apparatus consists in: strategies of relations of forces supporting, and supported by, types of knowledge.[114]

In summary, as I have established so far, the related crises over social media well-being, as expressed in psychologized, mediatized, marketized domains, has been configured as a crisis of user self-control.[115] The battle for social media well-being, in its current popular form, is therefore imagined, felt, and lived as a battle over individual habits. This can be understood as an operative form of neuroliberal governance, insofar as the impositions of behavioral change found in discourses of active, controlled use are responsive to historical problematics of (neo)liberal administration, market ideology, and the regulation of human freedom. User habits, therefore, are precisely what are at stake in the governmental functioning of social media well-being in the present day. Examining how habit is conceived, problematized, and administered in discourses and designs of social media well-being will thus sharpen my focus on the governance of social media well-being, opening up the issue onto more generative political, empirical, and theoretical grounds as a result.[116] The next sections will first detail how this effort can be empirically supported through select modes of sociotechnical inquiry, and then introduce how those modes will be employed throughout the following chapters in presenting the case study of Facebook.

Relational Habits and Sociotechnical Scripts

Moving beyond the idea that habits are immaculately controllable by the individual, habits have instead been viewed as the things that are formed when "socio-cultural and bio-physical" human elements interact with the lived environment.[117] Habits incorporate the outside in, as it were, linking individuals to the contexts of their existences, to the norms, values, hopes, and cultures of their environing world, as well as their own responses to them.[118] This relational view of habit has been used to sidestep the unproductive frameworks of user control and active/passive use that have commonly been used to discuss social media well-being to date. Thinkers such as Wendy Chun, for example, suggest that social media habits "move between the voluntary and the involuntary," conceptually troubling the idea that human beings can ever be fully in charge of the technologized worlds within which they live.[119] Such ideas echo Mariana Valverde's statement that habits are "precisely those patterns of action that are neither fully willed nor utterly determined," unsettling stable views of autonomy and undermining attempts to pin down human will and intention into an identifiable (limiting) form.[120]

Rather than users either controlling their habits of social media or being controlled by them, the inculcation of habit on social media instead operates as a process of complex and reciprocal environmental conditioning—which, as already mentioned, is reflective of, and formed through, shifting matrices of personal freedom and governance. The American philosopher of habit John Dewey, writing in the early twentieth century, was one of the first to recognize the technological constitution of this process. Dewey argues that all human activities, and the habits through which they become sedimented, occur within environments that depend on technology for their shape. He explains that technologies

> are actual means only when brought into conjunction with eye, arm and hand in some specific operation. And eye, arm and hand are, correspondingly, means proper only when they are in active operation. And whenever they are in action they are cooperating with external materials and energies. Without support from beyond themselves the eye stares blankly and the hand moves fumblingly. They are means only when they enter into organization with things which independently accomplish definite results.[121]

Dewey suggests that it is through these technological/human organizations that habits are formed, along with the possibilities of life they establish. As such, it is difficult to ascertain a strict ethical hierarchical chain in the formation of human action: who or what is responsible for habits, such as those formed on social media, is tricky to discern.

This insight has obvious parallels with actor-network theory (ANT), which explores the interrelated networks said to support nonhuman-human relations. For example, Bruno Latour, who is often affiliated with the ANT approach, writes that "there is no sense in which humans may be said to exist as humans without entering into commerce with what authorises and enables them to exist (i.e. to act)."[122] Here, Latour is referring to a process that he calls technical mediation—the idea that the possibility of all human activity is enmeshed with, and dependent on, the presence of objects. All life is technologically mediated, from objects as mundane as doors and speed bumps to extravagant processes of algorithmic decision-making.[123] Latour calls these varieties of objects *actors*, insofar as they work to facilitate, prompt, inhibit, or enable action in the world.[124] Paying attention to these nonhuman entities is, for Latour, to pay attention to the "missing masses" that ensure the abiding sequences of everyday life, sequences that set the scene for any human action, in any place, to occur at all.[125]

Habits are formed when humans come into a predictable and patterned relationship with embedded networks of human and nonhuman entities. Madeleine Akrich, a scholar of science and technology studies, argues that by arranging these relations, technologies can work to "stabilize, naturalize, depoliticize, and translate" social relations to such an extent that it can often appear as if there was "never any possibility it could have been otherwise" in the world.[126] For Akrich, the attempted stabilization of technical objects, who their ideal human users are, and the habits they have been designed to inculcate "is a process of reciprocal definition," whereby technologies "build our history . . . and impose certain frameworks" of appropriate human activity in their contexts of use.[127] Akrich employs a cinematic simile to describe this process, observing that "like a film script, technical objects define a framework of action together with the actors and the space in which they are supposed to act."[128] Latour relatedly discusses this process as "inscription," whereby "programs of action" are incorporated into the design of, and the discourse surrounding, particular technologies.[129] Some ANT approaches have been criticized for advocating a flat ontological perspective, perpetuating an apolitical approach to research that seeks to simply describe relationships of human/nonhuman actors.[130] However, in positioning actors in relation to each other, and by making certain courses of action more likely than others as a result, I argue that the scripting of technology can be similarly examined through analytics of power and governance.

In doing so, I build on the thought of software studies scholars Matthew Fuller and Andrew Goffey, who argue that technological scripts "regularise actions" by producing "enabled and entrained" users.[131] Through this process, scripts transmit and transform "operations and dynamics of power."[132] The idea of the sociotechnical script, as such, can be used to examine the stable "obduracy" of artifacts, while also capturing the relational dynamics that coproduce both users and those artifacts within the historical milieu of their inception and use—something Steve Woolgar describes as a process of *configuration*.[133] Script analysis, as investigations of this kind have been termed, examine the prescriptions of use built into technological products through empirical studies of their technical functions, the way these functions are advertised to intended users in particular consumer markets, and how these prescriptions play out in their actual human use in various environments.[134] Through a sustained case study of Facebook, this book will adopt and adapt similar frameworks of script analysis to examine how discourses of self-control and healthy habits are materially inscribed in designs of social media well-being, where these ideas come from, whose interests they serve, and how users themselves are reacting to and enacting them through their interactions with platforms.[135] The focus on Facebook, which to some readers may appear an outdated choice, follows Taina Bucher's invitation to study platforms beyond their relative position within fluctuating social media trends, instead examining their significance in wider terms: how they provide infrastructure for human sociality and identity, for example, or how they enable networked surveillance and globalized capitalist flows of data.[136] Thus, the empirical canvas of Facebook is stretched not as an end in itself, but rather as a means to explore enduring concerns about the nature of living well in digital spheres and, more fundamentally, what it means to constitute ourselves as thinking, feeling, and interacting humans in the world today.

Book Outline and Intentions

Building on the idea that health and well-being is a culturally and historically contingent state of existence, chapter 1 will examine the grounds upon which Facebook scripts its ideal healthy users, in relation to which bodies of knowledge, and with what implications. By analyzing Facebook's combined scientific and promotional discourses, where healthy active use is constructed and presented as the key to user well-being on the platform, I will show how Facebook's public relations materials—including official blogs, speeches, advertisements, and other gray media—rearticulate Facebook's funded social psychology and HCI research to establish its programs of living well online. Through a peculiar blend of evolutionary psychology and neoliberal theories of social capital, such research suggests that habits of active use are expressions of naturally occurring human drives. The findings of these studies are used to rhetorically justify the positioning of active use as the imagined cornerstone of user well-being on the platform, and have been used by Facebook to respond to the public criticism surrounding the psychological, political, technological, and cultural utility of its services. Such a scripting of the well-being hopes and risks of social media will be shown to operate through what Luke Stark has termed the *psycho-computational complex*— the generative imbrication between knowledge produced in psy-disciplines, computational designs, and social media business models.[137] In this way, the habits of ideal active use that Facebook recommends to its users will be examined as part of a strategy of power that at once makes its users visible and known as beings of a certain type, while also seeking to ensure Facebook's continued profitability as a capitalist data platform in the face of intense public scrutiny. From this, I will argue that critical researchers ought to be wary of engaging with concepts and measurements endorsed by platforms themselves, such as active use, which contain within them this strategic function. Instead, chapter 1 argues that researchers ought to create and apply new terms of analysis in the study of social media well-being, beyond those that simply buttress platforms' own interests.

Chapter 2 narrows its empirical focus to one aspect of Facebook's infrastructure, its Feed, in order to examine how Facebook's ideal active users are scripted in the design of the platform itself. It will examine how healthy users are technically administered online through the arrangement of freedom and choice, drawing attention to current ideologies of nudge present in HCI that imbue computational designers with the right to structure human behavior in certain directions, as opposed to others. Interestingly, in contrast to the findings of chapter 1, we will find that the way Facebook's Feed nudges its users toward healthy habits of use actually reveals a distrust in users' ability to act in their own best interests on the platform. Chapter 2 will examine the liberal paternalist roots and justifications of this designed distrust, showing how the Feed's nudge design aims to influence the behavioral decisions of users through intervening in "both the situations in which decisions are made and the emotional drivers of those decisions."[138] Overall, this chapter will position social media feeds as *neuroliberal interfaces* that govern their users "through the psychological appropriation of [digital] space"—raising questions about how user agency is administered on platforms today.[139] My argument in this chapter will thus expand the concept of neuroliberalism onto new empirical terrains, exploring the conceptual tensions between neoliberalism, freedom, and choice to be found therein, while offering new insights into the normative functioning of HCI and design that can be applied to other digital environments. In sum, who we trust to articulate and cultivate the digital good life will be up for debate in this chapter.

Chapter 3 will investigate how social media users are reacting to the contradictory scripting of healthy use in their interactions with platforms, by looking at how they respond to material discursive configurations of social media well-being in their daily lives. Drawing upon data from in-depth interviews with British Facebook users as we scrolled down their personal feeds together, I will reveal how participants spoke about their attempts to manage their use of social media as a losing battle of self-control. Primarily, users reflected upon the asymmetrical power relations involved in inhabiting an extractive platform environment designed to profit from their interactions with it. Despite participants' well-articulated rationales for their online struggles, which most notably revolved around the demands of the aforementioned attention economy, these users spoke about the ways in which failing to control their habits on the Feed (as they thought they should) produced painful feelings of internal guilt and public shame. This chapter will argue that the discursive repertoires employed by participants to discuss their well-being struggles with the Feed constitute tangible effects of responsibilization, revealing the presence of a normative (and diminished) neuroliberal form of life that structured how users felt they should communicate, reflect upon, and respond to their social media well-being habits in their everyday existence.

The conclusion of this book will reflect on the possibilities for change open to users in the face of the governance of well-being on social media. Chiefly, it will present the Foucauldian modes of critique employed in the preceding chapters as key tactics of refusal toward this end, showing how these modes of problematization operate as a "form of disassembly that productively opens the contingent present to an underdetermined future."[140] These possibilities will be shown to operate on the ontological terrain of the individual, whereby each user has the opportunity to clarify and objectify the discursive material modes through which they are constituted as healthy subjects in the present day. I will offer *counter-conduct* and *care of the self* as two potentially transformative forms of self-relation for users to explore in this regard, showing how they generate political and ethical dynamics able to disturb the ease with which current therapeutics of social media well-being are delivered and accepted. Through this, I will open the opportunity for a new ethic of living well with social media to emerge, beyond its current neuroliberal thresholds and technological administration, and its corresponding entanglement with responsibilized discourses of individualized well-being.

Overall, my study of the healthy social media user—how it is scripted in discourse and design and how people are relating to its force—aims to (1) understand how different human subjects are *made* through historical apparatuses of power, (2) analyze "the limits imposed on" these subjects in the process, and (3) "experiment with the possibility of going beyond" such limits through conceptual and empirical clarification.[141] Although a concern of several critical traditions, these interests have principally grown out of my engagement with Foucauldian poststructuralism, science and technology studies' focus on the configuration of users, the empirical concerns of disconnection studies, and my formative education in cultural studies. In respect to the latter, Stuart Hall's claim that "the only theory worth having is that which you have to fight off" inspires the analysis found in this book.[142] Such a fight does not seek definitive answers, but aims toward intellectual destabilization, breaching new interpretive thresholds that demand to be met on their own terms. Using this approach, I hope to show how presently felt digital norms can operate unchallenged only as long as their epistemological edifices remain intact, their axiological vanishing points remain unexposed, and their technological administration goes unchecked. Consequently, by the end of this book, the reader will be in a better position to critically assess whether the values, politics, and practices expressed through governance of well-being on social media are actually ones they wish to endorse and live by, or not.

1 *Healthy Use and How to Refuse It*

From a young age, we are taught that there are some things in life that are good for our health, and some things that are not. Eat your greens, a parent might once have said, and you'll grow up big and strong. Stop watching TV all day, or your eyes will go square. Manage your social media use, or your brain will fry. As we mature some of these suggestions stick, some don't. And when we venture further afield, simple comparisons with the people we meet show that not everyone's idea of healthy living is the same. A gym session at 4 a.m. may get the blood flowing for some. For others, nothing could be worse. Meditation could help positively balance a hectic schedule for a beleaguered worker. Another may simply be met with boredom and frustration.

A cursory glance through history further magnifies the discrepancies between different visions of health at different times and places. Since European antiquity, for example, and right up to the nineteenth century, bloodletting was prized as both a prophylactic and therapeutic practice.[1] In the sixteenth-century Ottoman Empire, health depended on fixed astrological readings.[2] And in ancient Mesopotamia, health was a reward for spiritual piety, illness a sign of moral destitution.[3] While perhaps strange to the contemporary reader, these ideas were not simply plucked from thin air at the time. As in the present day, historical therapies all mobilize certain beliefs, worldviews, and particular forms of expertise to ground their validity as health interventions. For example, the ancients viewed bloodletting as a way to balance the four elemental humors of the human body; according to the Roman-Greek physician Galen, blood is the most dominant humor and requires regular release.[4] Today, think of the different epistemic and axiological registers employed by various medical traditions, such as Western medicine, traditional Chinese medicine, or ayurveda, to diagnose and treat health and illness.[5] Whether scientifically, spiritually, or ecologically grounded, we can observe that different pathways toward health reveal themselves when viewed through different historico-cultural frameworks. Commitment to one or the other is required for any suggested health intervention to make sense for those involved.

While notions of health are always historical in character, all are similar insofar as the invocation of health at different times and places necessarily appeals to some form of justificatory architecture or another. This is good for you *because*; this is bad for you *because*; do this instead *because*. Writing in early twentieth-century France, the philosopher of science and physician Georges Canguilhem explored these justificatory relations. In particular, Canguilhem examined the ways in which Western ideas of health and disease are imbricated with corresponding ideas of the normal and pathological.[6] Canguilhem explored the idea that health on its own is "silent," and only comes forward in relation to the gripes and troubles of disease that deviate from it.[7] As such, health is not a concept of existence but rather a relational norm—a norm "whose function and value is to be brought into contact with existence in order to stimulate modification."[8] Extrapolating further, Canguilhem shows that health, "as a norm, or rule," and following its Latin root *norma* (T-square), "is what can be used to right, to square, to straighten."[9]

Norms, therefore, like concepts of health, function to constrain existence. Canguilhem writes: "To set a norm (*normer*), to normalise, is to impose a requirement on an existence, a given whose variety, disparity, with regard to the requirement, present themselves as a hostile, even more than an unknown, indeterminant. . . . The concept of right, depending on whether it is a matter of geometry, morality or technology, qualifies what offers resistance to its application of twisted, crooked or awkward."[10] In this way, as Foucault (who was Canguilhem's student) went on to examine, and as Nikolas Rose has explored vis-à-vis more recent developments in molecular biopolitics, health designates a normative relation between acceptable and unacceptable states of being, between ideal modes of existence and their opposite.[11] All of this combined offers versions of life to strive toward and those to avoid. When we come across suggestions of healthy living, like the styles of healthy technological engagement offered up by social media companies today, therefore, we are unavoidably entering into a game of norms. Because of this, we are also entering into relations of power.

This chapter will explore the processes of configuration through which Facebook constructs modes of ideal, healthy, normal use, as well as its corresponding ideal healthy user. Inspired by the style of Foucauldian analytics of power established in the introduction, the scripting of these users will be understood as a form of contemporary subjectivation, whereby individuals are led to imagine and relate to themselves as beings with certain characteristics, capacities, desires, proclivities, and natures. Additionally, we will explore how agentic activity upon these self-interpretations also serves the interests of particular institutions. In this case, by presenting well-being online solely as an outcome of user activity—itself an outcome of user choice—Facebook's vision of healthy active use offers a path to well-being for Facebook users to willfully follow on the platform. Importantly, following this path is framed as if it were in users' own interests to do so. These actions also function strategically in Facebook's economic favor by maintaining profitable avenues of datafication on the platform. That is, healthy active use on platforms generates more data for Facebook to extract and sell to interested third parties, leading to the accrual of more value for the company and its shareholders.

Accordingly, this chapter argues that discourses of healthy active use serve a vital purpose within the governance of well-being on social media. Recalling a concept coined by Tuomo Tiisala that I introduced in the introduction, I will argue that Facebook's attempt to align the interests of its business with the well-being interests of its users *topically excludes* any critical consideration of either Facebook's computationally persuasive capitalist functioning or how the platform effectively *mediates* the activity it enables.[12] Moreover, through the narrow behavioral parameters of individual active use that Facebook promotes as the key to well-being online, we are also made blind to the wider *social determinants of health* that unevenly impact users prior to and during their interactions with platforms.

To establish these arguments, I will examine the publicly available promotional materials and scientific research released by Facebook to outline its original formulation of ideal healthy active use in the late 2010s. Such ideas were first introduced to public audiences in the aftermath of Facebook's embroilment in the Cambridge Analytica scandal, and Mark Zuckerberg's widely publicized hearing in front of the US legislature in 2018 concerning Facebook's business operations. While Facebook has continued to publish research on well-being in more recent years, returning to these original documents will allow us to examine the operation of a particular *psycho-computational complex* extant at its moment of inception. Here, following Luke Stark, we will see how knowledge from the psy-disciplines, computational design, and social media business models all combine within Facebook's discourse of healthy use.[13] This works to shape user behavior in certain directions, while also seeking to constrain public and personal interpretations of this behavior in terms agreeable to Facebook itself.

Overall, this chapter begins an exploration of Facebook's version of transparent "corporate authenticity," arguing that Facebook's early efforts to pin down what well-being means on the platform sought to limit the field of possible interpretations of its psychological, political, technological, and cultural utility at a time of potential destabilization.[14] In Foucauldian terms, we can view these attempts as part of a discursive material *apparatus* formed in response to an "urgent need"—specifically Facebook's need to assuage user (and shareholder) doubt about its social, cultural, and political value in the world.[15] This chapter, then, is concerned with the ways in which Facebook's discourse of well-being addresses the public criticism of its "toxic" services in a way that both secures its economic functioning and erects a regime of healthy normality for users to situate themselves within and compare themselves against. A heady concoction, certainly, and one that I will do my best to distill into something intelligible below.

Psycho-computational Rhetorics of Justification

According to Madeleine Akrich, whose notion of the sociotechnical script methodologically grounds the empirical analysis of this book, the designers and purveyors of technologies (like social media) incorporate a "vision of (or prediction about) the world in the technical content" of the object itself, as well as in the communication materials surrounding their promotion.[16] These visions, for Akrich, construct the perceived needs of certain user groups while often misrepresenting or altogether neglecting others.[17] Else Rommes, for instance, suggests that technical scripts "attribute and delegate specific competencies, actions, and responsibilities to their envisioned users," arguing that assumptions about users and use-context are materialized in discourse and design.[18] These ideas build on the work of STS scholar Steve Woolgar, who shows how the creators, designers, and marketers of technologies "attempt to define and delimit the user's possible actions" through their technical affordances and broader promotional paratext.[19] Rather than the user existing a priori to a technology's release, "by setting parameters for the user's actions," Woolgar suggests, "the evolving machine effectively attempts to configure the user."[20] This means that a given technology and its dissemination relay "basic assumptions" about both its ideal purpose and how that purpose can fulfill the imagined needs of its ideal users.[21]

The design and promotional discourses of technological products generate technological scripts that communicate limited worldviews and curtailed models of usership. Bryan Pfaffenberger, for example, argues that artifacts are always "projected into a spatially defined, discursively regulated social context" by their creators, who seek to restrict and stabilize the many potential interpretations of their social role, value, and use in the world.[22] Relatedly, Helen Nissenbaum writes that the producers of technological products are necessarily engaged in the task of describing how their "technology links into and satisfies certain cultural or symbolic needs that people have."[23] Designed configurations of ideal human users and technical objects, therefore, represent political circumscriptions of the world by establishing and expressing both how they ought to be used and by whom. The sociotechnical dramas within which Facebook most forcefully projects its vision of ideal healthy use respond to the psychological controversies that have historically surrounded its services. As outlined in the introduction, these involve the observable propensity for increased social media use to be positively correlated with poor mental health outcomes, such as depression and anxiety.

These issues came to a head on April 10, 2018, during Zuckerberg's appearance before the US Senate's Committee on Commerce, Science, and Transportation, where the sociopolitical value of Facebook was being publicly reevaluated in the highest echelons of government. The hearing followed several high-profile political scandals involving the platform, including nefarious campaign activity during the 2016 presidential election. Most notably, Russian agents were found spreading misinformation on Facebook, and the private political consultancy firm Cambridge Analytica had pursued psychologized micro-campaigns targeting local users in swing states.[24] Meanwhile, the platform was widely criticized for creating a toxic social environment linked to worsening mental health. Whether or not Facebook contributed to the well-being of users, and society at large, was increasingly a matter for debate.

In response to repeated questioning about these key issues, Zuckerberg claimed he viewed Facebook's "responsibility as not just building services that people like, but building services that are good for people and good for society as well."[25] While this seems fairly innocuous, such statements are, in fact, doing a lot of heavy lifting. As Judith Butler reminds us, references to the social good ought not to be taken at face value. Rather, they should be examined as prompts for existential questioning, revelatory of core values, morals, and habits. For Butler, "If I ask how best to live, or how to lead a good life, I seem to draw upon not only ideas of what is good, but also of what is living, and what is life. I must have a sense of my life in order to ask what kind of life to lead, and my life must appear to me as something I might lead, something that does not just lead me."[26] When we encounter questions of the human good, and how it should be lived, we are faced with questions of personal agency, with how best to exercise our freedom in the hope of reaching optimum states of being. In this way, while potentially helping individuals orient themselves toward styles of life that work for them, discourses of the good life can also be put to work in processes of governance, which seek to shape human behavior in particular directions, for particular ends. Because discourses of the good life furnish people with a reason to act, as if it were in their own interests to do so, they can be disseminated and promoted by particular actors hoping to conduct the conduct of others for strategic purposes.[27]

To establish particular Facebook activities as being "good" for humans is to mobilize particular accounts of human wants and needs. In other words, it is to mobilize particular accounts of human nature. As shown in the introduction, what counts as the human good, and the corresponding visions of well-being that accompany it, necessarily relay and reinforce the specific interests of those wishing to set certain forms of life in motion. These configurations include some while working to exclude and discriminate against many others. Contingent values, beliefs, and norms are mobilized whenever the good life is articulated to justify certain political, economic, and health interventionist practices at different moments. Hence, alarm bells should ring when we hear Facebook's CEO talk about individual and societal good as a motivation for how they build their commercial services.

However, as we will see throughout this chapter, Facebook buttresses its contingent visions of user well-being by invoking psychological knowledge as its scientific foundation. In particular, Facebook's leaders, advertisements, and user guides all construct a shared idea of the good active user in relation to findings emerging from psychology and the field of human-computer interaction (HCI), most notably from studies undertaken by Facebook's own or affiliated researchers. Through these invocations, Facebook presents its well-being interventions in the lives of users as necessary and valid, insofar as they are based on seemingly objective scientific measures. Luke Stark has previously examined similar imbrications between the psychological sciences, computational practice, and social media design as part of a *psycho-computational complex*, whereby the vast and ubiquitous personal data extracted from social media platforms can be used to target and administer individual behavior on a massive scale.[28]

However, as Nikolas Rose states, the psycho-computational aspect of Facebook's apparatus of user well-being can also be understood as "part of the history of the ways in which human beings have regulated others and have regulated themselves in the light of certain games of truth."[29] Specifically, the interrelated practices of testing, measuring, scoring, ranking, and comparing found in the psychological studies of user well-being invoked by Facebook make its users "intelligible and practicable" subjects, ripe for intervention.[30] By virtue of this—by being assessed and known in this way—psychologized human beings, such as Facebook's users, are rendered eminently *governable*.

Users' *governability* should be understood not only as how they are targeted through the workings of governments and political institutions, but also in the Foucauldian sense of the conduct of conduct—how institutions, individuals, and groups act "upon the actions of others in order to achieve certain ends."[31] For Rose, "The perspective of government draws our attention to all those multitudinous programs, proposals, and policies that have attempted to shape the conduct of individuals—not just to control, subdue, discipline, normalise, or reform them, but also to make them more intelligent, wise, happy, virtuous, healthy, productive, docile, enterprising, fulfilled, self-esteeming, empowered."[32] Modes of positive psychological invocation, of the kind practiced by Facebook, and as explored below, can encourage pathways of individual conduct as it were in the individuals' own benefit to follow them, all the while simultaneously ensuring that the profitable arrangement of Facebook's datafied business model will flourish. This is the generative, stabilizing dimension of power in action.

Active Use

Mark Zuckerberg's Senate testimony in April 2018, in which he qualifies his statements concerning the good use of the platform quoted above, provides an example of the psycho-computational complex in full effect:

> We study a lot of effects of well-being of our tools. . . . What we find in general is that you're using social media in order to build relation-ships, right? So, if you're sharing content with friends, you're inter-acting, then that is associated with all of the long-term measures of well-being that you'd intuitively think of: long-term health, long-term happiness, long-term feeling connected, feeling less lonely. But if you're using the internet and social media primarily to just passively consume content, and you're not engaging with other people, then it doesn't have those positive effects and it could be negative.[33]

There are plenty of assumptions in play here. Is active use really why users go on Facebook? And how can Zuckerberg know that doing so is "good" for their well-being? However, because Zuckerberg invokes Facebook's "study" of well-being to verify these claims, these ques-tions appear to have a reasonable answer: it's all research based. As such, the audience is asked to interpret active use as a recommenda-tion formed through and grounded in response to objective knowl-edge, imbuing Facebook's well-being interventions with a semblance of scientific validity as a result. Facebook's ideas of well-being appear to be evidence based and, as such, become harder to contest.

Frances Haugen's revelations in late 2021 lifted the lid on Face-book's research into user mental health on the platform, yet Face-book cannot really be accused of shyness in presenting its research to public audiences. In fact, Facebook frequently refers to its own re-search to justify its interventions in the everyday lives of its billions of users. For instance, around the time of Zuckerberg's congressional hearings, Chris Cox, then head of product at Facebook, in an inter-view with *Wired* magazine, suggested that people want to have conversations [on Facebook]. They don't want to be passively consuming content. This is connected with the research on well-being, which says that if you go somewhere and you just sit there and watch, and you don't talk to anybody, it can be sad. If you go to the same place and you have five or six conversations that are good around what's going on in the world, what you care about, you feel better.[34]

Similarly, in a speech at Morgan Stanley, also in 2018, Sheryl Sandberg, then chief operating officer of Facebook, claimed that "not all interactions in social media are equally good for people in terms of their psychological well-being," likewise engaging in scientific modes of veriction and echoing the hierarchy of activity espoused by Zuckerberg and Cox above.[35] Elsewhere, Adam Mosseri, then head of Facebook's News Feed, spoke at length about healthy active Facebook use and well-being in a presentation at Facebook's 2018 F8 developer conference, using Facebook's own research to ground suggestions that the News Feed has been designed to inculcate good active social habits in users over deleterious ones.[36]

The psychological justifications and discursive opposition of *active* and *passive* use found in these statements and others can thus be identified as patterns in the well-being discourses adopted by Facebook's leaders in early 2018. Implicitly, the choice between these two modes of activity is presented as a better or worse health decision by the user: active use is good, passive use is bad. Facebook thus constructs a normative vision of its ideal healthy user, laying out a particular path toward the digital good life for the user to follow, seemingly established through scientific means.

Monetizing Natural Needs

Facebook originally presented the psychological evidence behind its endorsement of active use in a public-facing blog series called *Hard*

Questions. According to Facebook, *Hard Questions* was intended to make its services "more open and accountable."[37] This could be deemed necessary in the face of the aforementioned criticisms increasingly leveled at the platform in the mid- to late 2010s. The blog series, for instance, offers insight into how Facebook publicly conceptualizes and presents its actions on various sociopolitical issues, addressing topics such as extremist activity on Facebook, fake news, data privacy, and democracy. The blog post that first addresses user well-being at length is titled "Is Spending Time on Social Media Bad for Us?" and is credited to David Ginsberg, then director of research, and Moira Burke, then a social psychologist at Facebook.[38] The company's well-being research that Ginsberg and Burke present suggests that how people choose to use social media determines the extent to which it is a positive or negative force in their lives. In this blog, Facebook is attempting to stage the psycho-computational crisis of social media well-being in its own terms, gathering selected information and materials to fuse into a topical narrative, and inviting its users to relate to their online habits in preconfigured ways. We can usefully understand this as a form of performative corporate responsibility, a process of "proprietorial enframing" whereby companies seek to preempt and curtail any potential criticisms of their business practices through their own funded research, PR, public statements, self-regulation, and philanthropic endeavors.[39]

The blog begins by acknowledging the psychological issues that can arise through engagement with the platform, including increased social isolation, negative social comparison, and anxiety. However, foreshadowing the statements by Facebook's leaders quoted above, Ginsberg and Burke write: "According to the research, it really comes down to how you use the technology. For example, on social media, you can passively scroll through posts, much like watching TV, or actively interact with friends—messaging and commenting on each other's posts. Just like in person, interacting with people you care about can be beneficial, while simply watching others from the sidelines may make you feel worse."[40] The blog presents findings from particular psychological studies to bolster these claims ("the research"), especially those that examine the psychological impact of Facebook through the binary of active/passive use. These studies seem to show that measures of well-being can increase if Facebook users engage in certain active habits—such as private messaging, liking photos, and commenting—as opposed to passive habits like scrolling down the feed without interacting with posts or failing to message friends and family.

The blog connects this particular view of user well-being to one of Facebook's first psychological studies on the issue, coauthored by Burke and Robert E. Kraut.[41] This piece of research is front and center of Facebook's public relations discourse of active/passive use in the mid- to late 2010s, and thus represents a crucial site of analysis for this chapter. However, before I turn to this and related research, it is important to repeat a key point that I made in the introduction concerning how I will handle these sources. My analysis of these psychological and HCI studies does not engage in a critique of their findings in terms of their reproducibility, methodological validity, or empirical salience. Rather, my task involves carefully analyzing how the image of Facebook's ideal user is formed through the specific mobilization of certain ideas of human nature, health, well-being, conduct, agency, and action. This effort sets the ground for an exploration of how these ideas join up with other elements of Facebook's PR strategy to produce a grid of intelligibility through which users are led to understand certain modes of Facebook activity as *good* for them to adopt, and others as activities they should avoid. This is not to say that these connected visions are either true or false; rather, it is intended to show how they are necessarily constructed, while highlighting how they function within scripted regimes of social media governance and normalization.

What is more, it is not my claim that these effects are singularly *intentional*. Instead, I hope to highlight the ways power, knowledge, and topical exclusion combine, often without any one directing force or intentionality, to set certain styles of life in action as opposed to others. In particular, building on the work of Susan Oman, examining how well-being is constructed as a measurable, categorizable phenomenon in these studies can reveal implicit norms and assumptions behind ostensibly neutral well-being data.[42] Hence, exposing these assumptions to critical consideration will allow us to examine the workings of the psycho-computational complex in more detail, offering a clearer understanding of whether Facebook's program of healthy active use, as well as its effects, is actually something we wish to endorse ourselves—as individuals and as scholars.

In Burke and Kraut's paper on the relationship between types of use and user well-being, which is at the heart of Facebook's vision of active/passive use, they argue that Facebook exists as a neutral tool that could benefit users' well-being if used in a proactive manner. The core argument that holds this work together is grounded in evolutionary psychology, building "upon the assumption that people benefit from social interaction with others," writing that "humans are a social species, with many survival advantages accruing from our connections to others."[43] In particular, this assumption is bolstered by a reference to Roy Baumeister and Mark Leary's evolutionary concept of human belonging.[44] This view posits that humans have evolved to be reciprocally caring and social creatures in order to maintain evolutionary advantages in potentially threatening environments. On social media, the argument follows, the positive emotional ties that bind humans with others in familial groups, friendship networks, and romantic relationships are said to be distinct characteristics that grant access to reproductive mates, mutual protection, and resources such as shelter and food. Relatedly, this theory suggests that human empathy and communication, of the kind said to be enabled by Facebook, developed as evolutionary and physiological necessities of human survival. By engaging with these ideas, Facebook's researchers are drawing upon evolutionary discourses to naturalize active use of the platform. As such, the types of active communications supported by Facebook are imagined by its researchers as supporting innate human proclivities and natural evolutionary needs.

Once situated in this way, this type of Facebook activity can be neatly fitted within a recognizable evolutionary lineage. Snugly positioned as part of humankind's biological development, we are led to view active Facebook use as a naturally occurring phenomenon. This is a persuasive move and serves an invaluable strategic function for Facebook. Principally, as a result of this positioning, the ways in which Facebook's design actually prompts users toward a particular type of branded social activity for a primary capitalist purpose are reframed. Facebook's evolutionary narrative effectively presents its harvesting of user data as a happy byproduct of its platform servicing natural human needs.

Essentially, Facebook monetizes its services by collecting and selling data generated by user activity. By tracking all of its users' profiles, interactions, relationships, comments, likes, shares, and private messages, Facebook constructs an image of their cultural interests, relationship status, education, geographic location, the organizations and networks they are affiliated with, their scrolling activity, time spent on pages, and so on.[45] By aggregating the data from each profile and its associated social networking activity, Facebook produces highly granular data on each of its users. From these data imprints, demographics of age, gender, sexual orientation, class, ethnicity, and myriad other categories can be approximated through a wide-scale comparison of all Facebook users and their respective activities. These various attributes of user identity and predicted preferences can then be sold as customized data sets by Facebook to advertisers (commercial, political, or otherwise) seeking to target particular demographics of users on the platform (and at other locations on the internet and beyond) with quasi-personalized messaging. On the basis of these demographic groupings, which advertisers can further modify and categorize in relation to their specific goals and commercial aims, different groups of users are targeted with different advertisements at different times—through a variety of means, in a variety of locations.

In Marxist terms, communicative activity on commercial social media like Facebook, therefore, can be understood as *digital labor*, insofar as it produces a digital commodity (data) that creates use-value for those that own it (platforms).[46] Users are not paid for this labor, so the data they produce can be considered *surplus value*. The ostensible benefits users receive from their engagements with social media—chatting with friends, commenting on entertaining memes, and so on—put a positive sheen on this arrangement, despite its essentially exploitative economic character. On this, Christian Fuchs writes: "Users are productive consumers who produce commodities and profit—their user labour is exploited. But this exploitation does not feel like toil, it is rather more like play and takes place during leisure time outside of wage labour—it is unpaid labour and play labour."[47] Beyond any corporate messaging about building products that are "good for people and good for society," following digital culture scholars Cristina Alaimo and Jannis Kallinikos, we should therefore not forget that Facebook constructs the conditions of user interactions exclusively for the extraction of surplus value.[48] Moreover, rather than existing prior to their engagement with the platform, Facebook users, as datafied bundles of clicks, interactions, and predicted preferences, are instead created as "social objects" on the platform.[49] That is, the digitized behaviors tracked and measured by Facebook, Alaimo and Kallinikos argue, would not exist "outside the engineered context" of the platform itself.[50] Instead, the types of social interactions made possible by Facebook, as well as the wider net-worked social groups they support, are better considered as the re-sult of a "designed sociality" that only serves to produce users as "quantitative derivations of an engineered experience," working as a distinctly capitalist function.[51] This is as far away from user behavior online being a "natural" phenomenon as possible.

In referencing the work of evolutionary psychologists such as Baumeister and Leary, by contrast, Facebook and its researchers carve out a particular presentation of the Facebook user as an inher-ently social animal—a being whose healthy internal psyche and phys-ical vitality are linked to certain forms of sociality with other like creatures on the platform. In this way, Facebook naturalizes its users as social animals, who are said to *need* Facebook in order to flourish in their natural capacity as evolutionarily ordained communal be-ings. What is crucial for us here is how the supposedly inherent so-ciality of Facebook's ideal user is used to justify Facebook's recom-mendations for active, profitable use online. In this framework, adopting good Facebook habits of active, frequent communication is to act upon one's own innate human sociality. Here we can observe the way that active (economically valuable) use is presented as the key not only to living well as a Facebook user, but also to living well as a fully realized human being.

At this point, it is worthwhile to recall that determining what counts as beneficial human activity is related to the philosophical at-tempt to discern what it means to live well as a human in time, known as *eudaimonic well-being*.[52] In this way, Facebook and its team of re-searchers are involved in an inherently normative task. Philosopher of well-being Philippa Foot writes that "to determine what is good-ness and defect of character, disposition, and choice, we must consider what human good is and how human beings live: in other words, what kind of living thing a human being is."[53] Facebook seems to wager that it doesn't really matter to its user audience that the company is making money off their activities, as those users are simply fulfilling an innate need for connection and desire to scroll. Personal data in exchange for the chance to flourish in your true capacity as a social human—a small price to pay, right?

The more user activity on the platform, the more data produced, the more Facebook can profit. Encouraging active use, therefore, works in Facebook's economic interest. And this core operation isn't something that Facebook shirks away from. For example, in the PR materials accompanying the reordering of the News Feed algorithm in 2018, Mosseri, as head of News Feed, claimed that Facebook's drive toward active use will benefit both users' well-being and Facebook's business model of data-driven targeted advertising.[54] Mosseri takes ownership of this fact, promoting active use "not only because we believe it's the right thing [for user well-being], but also because it's good for our business." Moreover, in an accompanying Facebook post, Zuckerberg explained that cultivating increased activity on the platform was "the right thing" for Facebook both ethically and economically, being "good for our community and our business over the long term."[55] Here, the interests of the user are presented as synonymous with the business interests of Facebook: a healthy user is an active user is a profitable user.

This serves as an example of what Michelle Murphy refers to as the "economization of life," whereby what feels like healthy, living social connection for users simultaneously works as an exploitative process that greases the cogs of continued digital capitalist expansion.[56] Through this lens, users imagining their exploited labor online as good for them simply masks the unpaid origin of their own subordination; active time spent on Facebook directly implicates the user with the dominating processes of primitive accumulation that keep unequal class structures in place.[57] Facebook's social media services, rather than being viewed as designed tools of capitalist value extraction, are instead said to work for the inherent interests of users by providing valuable, and (supposedly) necessary, spaces of social connection. As a result of this, the important questions surrounding the effects of Facebook's capitalist engineering of communication remain unasked. What is even more concerning, however, is that if we adopt the readymade interpretation of active healthy use provided to us by Facebook, the value of even considering those questions is undermined. Accepting Facebook's own terms of well-being thus represents a foreclosure of critique, and is something that critical researchers should seek to refuse at any given opportunity as a result.

Healthy Tools of Civilization

It is clear that we should be skeptical of the attempt to restrict our interpretations and analysis of social media well-being to the simplistic planes of active/passive use. Technologies like Facebook do not exist as empty intermediaries for willful, natural, human action. They are not simply wielded. They are better understood, following Bruno Latour, as key *actors* that *mediate* the activity that occurs through them, creating the very possibility for action to occur in the first place.[58] As such, to distinguish uses of inanimate technologies as "natural" or "willful" is a misnomer; technology and their users are mutually constitutive, and agency is shared between its human and nonhuman counterparts. Consequently, if we accept that users are effectively *configured*, made, by technologies and the discourses that surround them, to distinguish particular uses of Facebook—such as engaging in active use for social purposes—as natural inevitabilities is a major error. Nevertheless, despite these insights, Facebook continues to present its services as inanimate tools to be utilized by human subjects for their own evolutionary ends—a neutral technology that facilitates preexisting human tendencies to communicate, socialize, and connect with others online.

Because they allow users to cultivate social bonds with other humans, Facebook's services are afforded a high ethical value. These bonding processes are understood by Facebook's researchers in terms of "relationship maintenance" and "relational investment."[59] *Relationship maintenance* involves looking after one's social ties through regular interactions and communication. *Relational investment*, on the other hand, refers to the "symbolic value" of those communications, "independent of the content exchanged."[60] In this latter process, it is the frequency, length, and general effort involved in communication practices that matter. How this links to the natural evolutionary development of humankind is once again reiterated by Burke and Kraut, with another reference to evolutionary psychologists. This time, the authors invoke the work of Sam Roberts and Robin Dunbar, which argues that regular and repeated interpersonal communications are necessary to maintain both primate and human social networks.[61]

Burke and Kraut refer to this relationship maintenance as an "investment" of time and energy.[62] This focus on social investment is crucial: the extent to which relationships on Facebook benefit each user is said to correlate with the personal costs of time and energy put into them. Facebook's researchers bolster this argument through a reference to research emerging from social psychology, which suggests that high effort in *relationship maintenance* practices online, communications with friends for instance, can be associated with higher levels of social capital and well-being.[63] Social capital can be understood as the access to emotional and material resources that relationships in social networks can provide.[64] In its psychological construction, and as mobilized by Facebook, therefore, the more social ties one cultivates, the higher social capital one yields, the more resources one can access, the greater the well-being. Here, individual user well-being is pegged to the quality, scale, and usefulness of the resources that can be accessed in their social networks.

Upon this basis, the value of relationships in Facebook's construction of social well-being is essentially established through the prism of self-interest. We will come back to this pivotal idea in the following section. For now, let us follow the idea that healthy social media use exists as part of the linear development of self-interested human nature to other materials found on the *Hard Questions* blog that has anchored this investigation so far. On this blog, we further encounter a video titled "Social Media and Well-Being," which shares Facebook's research on the topic with a public audience in cartoon form. It begins with an illustrated representation of the globe zooming into a colorful and aesthetically simplified vision of civilized human social relations.[65] Reiterating the statements found in Facebook's study of well-being outlined above, the video begins with a voiceover instructing the viewer that "people have always been social animals. From hunting as a party, to forming tribes and laying the groundwork for civilization, humans have embraced the company of others." Cartoon representations of Neolithic tribal life, replete with spears and open fires, then seamlessly morph into representations of present-day humans scrolling on their phones. Comments, likes, and emojis are exchanged from one to the other in a visual representation of networked communication. People share, like, and interact through the tools of social media. In this way, the digital tribe emerges, with the evolutionary moral imperative of active use made real in cartoon form. Confirming this evolutionary narrative, the voiceover then suggests that "with today's digital tools, we're able to fulfill more of our social needs with the click of a button or tap on our phones." This makes a direct link between the evolution of the social human being and contemporary forms of online communication.

The sequential progress from the primordial tribe to Facebook's online social network reinforces the idea that the platform's continued global expansion follows a naturally ordained path. Facebook's services are said to be fulfilling innate human needs and can therefore be presented as universally and equally valuable to any potential human user on earth as a result. One way we can think of this globalizing, totalizing narrative is through the concept of the *coloniality of power*, which has examined how the calculative classification of healthy and unhealthy habits in colonial regimes, which constitute some styles of human existence as more natural than others, have been used within hierarchical tools of cultural differentiation and segmentation.[66] In particular, this draws from the work of Aníbal Quijano, who shows how the rendering of human types, human health, and human well-being—most notably in relation to designations of race—was created to justify both the actual and the epistemological violence wrought by modern colonial systems of European conquest and "civilized" social administration.[67] While not equivalent to these practices, Facebook's attempted interpretive control over what constitutes "good" use of its services, for whom, and why, follows similar epistemological and justificatory pathways.[68] That is, Facebook's attempt to construct a lineage within which every human on the planet can classify and understand themselves works to flatten alternative ways to imagine human life, and what is important to it, while simultaneously splitting behavior into healthy/unhealthy, good/bad, civilized/uncivilized binaries in the process. As such, Facebook's teleological account of evolutionary human flourishing and user well-being—one expressed in speeches, blog posts, and videos—positions the platform as a tool that can strengthen and maintain the social bonds necessary for continued human development, despite accusations of the contrary that were being leveled at the time of its release.[69]

The discursive statements collated on the *Hard Questions* blog concerning user well-being presented above, from psychological research to cartoon videos, although disparate, can be analyzed as part of a "unity of distribution" that conditions the "field of possible options" within which we are directed to think about and understand

Facebook's social value in the world.[70] Taken together, we can see how Facebook's discourse of well-being aims to produce a grid of intelligibility through which users are led to understand themselves, and their activity, as manifestations of a certain social essence. I have shown why we should refuse these easy interpretations: simply approaching social media in the terms that companies themselves define can say nothing about the way the discourses surrounding, and technical designs of, social media actually coproduce styles of human life, and for what purposes, in the present age. Meekly accepting Facebook use as a natural extension of human activity serves to obscure the very real ways such activity supports capitalist apparatuses of value extraction and colonial forms of epistemic totalization. When habitual Facebook use is rendered as an expression of innate social human being, it becomes very difficult to understand Facebook as anything other than a neutral arbiter of human sociality, despite there being nothing neutral, natural, or indeed inevitable about the style of social networking inculcated by social media companies like Facebook in the present day.

Self-Interested Sociality

In other locations within its well-being discourse, Facebook has published HCI research that can further reveal the shape of its ideal healthy users. Following Phoebe Sengers and colleagues, turning to these resources can help demonstrate the way HCI research implicitly and explicitly configures assumed users in technical systems.[71] "The design decisions" that HCI papers propose contain "values and assumptions" that purport certain worldviews, modes of interaction, and ideal users—all at the expense of others.[72] The recommendation of possible actions through computational design thus presupposes both the value of those actions and users capable of enacting them. Research emerging from HCI often functions to justify the design decisions taken by technology companies, whether research-ers themselves intended their work to be utilized as such or not.[73] As such, the way the knowledge produced in HCI research papers is used to justify Facebook's well-being interventions constitutes an ex-plicit operation of the psycho-computational complex, and espe-cially the functioning of power/knowledge within processes of gov-ernance.[74] Put simply, by presenting active use as the pathway to user flourishing online, and backing this up with HCI research, Face-book's discourse of well-being works to set certain styles of econom-ically valuable user activity in motion (power) through an appeal to scientific findings (knowledge). This section will trace the construc-tion of Facebook's vision of self-interested sociality to be found else-where in its HCI research, and explore how this merges with Face-book's view of natural use that I have examined above. I hope to show that when we pause and linger on how interested parties are conceiv-ing, measuring, and constructing well-being, and how subsequent data on well-being are invoked to validate, normalize, and justify cer-tain behavioral interventions in the everyday lives of people, as well as interpret their effects, we may find points of contestation that would have otherwise slipped below our consideration.

In Facebook's early HCI papers on well-being, the cultivation of social capital is rendered as the chief contributing factor to living well on the platform.[75] *Social capital*, in these studies, refers to the per-sonal "benefits made possible by the existence of a social struc-ture."[76] For Facebook's affiliated researchers, social capital is split into bridging and bonding social capital, and it is argued that in-creased access to both these kinds of social capital leads to improved measures of well-being. Mark Granovetter's work on the efficacy of "strong" and "weak" tie contacts forms the basis of this distinction.[77] Granovetter suggests that when looking for employment, the ability to mobilize the full range of one's extended social network (beyond immediate family) is a key predictor of success. *Bridging social capital* refs to weak-tie relationships that individuals maintain with distant contacts, and measures the support of a wider social network that can facilitate the formation of fresh ties in new situations of need. *Bonding social capital*, on the other hand, refers to the beneficial effects of deeper levels of personal relationships held between close ties in close-knit communities, and measures the support offered in the relationships found in the family or between longstanding work colleagues.

In the first of its papers on social capital and well-being, Facebook's affiliated researchers used server logs to collect activity data for 1,193 Facebook users over two months, which were then compared with survey results that assessed three related measures of well-being: bridging social capital, bonding social capital, and loneliness. In this study, levels of bridging social capital were assessed in participants' responses to statements such as "I come in contact with new people all the time," given on a five-point Likert scale ranging from strongly disagree to strongly agree. Participants' bonding social capital was measured through similarly graded responses to items such as "There are several people I trust to help solve my problems." Finally, loneliness was assessed using eight items taken from the UCLA loneliness scale.[78] The combined scores of these three measures resulted in a score of overall well-being for each participant. The various types of Facebook activity scraped from the server logs of each participant were then compared with respective well-being scores.

From the results of these tests, forms of directed communication, such as private messaging and commenting on statuses, were associated with improved levels of bonding social capital, overall user well-being, and lower reported loneliness. Resonant with Facebook's social psychology outlined above, the value of direct forms of communication was said to lie in their ability to increase the channels of emotional support open to users at any given time. This notion was used to explain how lower feelings of loneliness and greater feelings of social support were linked to active use. Conversely, consumptive activity, such as passively observing interactions on Facebook, led to a reduction in levels of bridging social capital and increased feelings of loneliness. The study characterized the value of one-to-one conversations with close ties on Facebook as investments in bonding social capital, which is said to naturally lead to higher levels of user well-being. In opposition, passive interactions were presented as damaging to bridging social capital and were instead linked with lower levels of well-being and feelings of loneliness.

Elsewhere in its HCI research on well-being, Facebook similarly and repeatedly characterizes relationships as investments in social capital. For instance, in a follow-up study on this initial work on social capital and well-being, investing time and energy into relationships is said to constitute healthy Facebook practice by ensuring that social ties remain intact over time.[79] These social investments are characterized as increasing the likelihood that social resources will be available to users if needed later down the line. In this model, the rational motivation for ideal healthy usership on Facebook is the expected return individuals would gain on their emotional investment in others in the future. Once viewed in combination with Facebook's evolutionary discourse, these localized (Western) imaginations of social investment become naturalized as universal user characteristics.

Neoliberal Social Capital

In its studies on user well-being and social capital, Facebook positions its services as naturally good for users upon a very narrow conceptualization of user well-being that is pegged to a distinct form of equivalized self-interested sociality. To understand why and how this view percolates through Facebook's thinking on the topic, and why we would do well to challenge it, we must understand the pervasive cultural, social, and political logics it draws upon. As outlined in the introduction, this requires an engagement with the neoliberal milieu within which Facebook has risen to global significance. Examining the explicitly political constitution of Facebook's healthy user will add yet another element to the psycho-computational complex at the heart of discourses and designs of active use, thus deepening our interpretation of its contemporary operation and spread.

Again, following Foucault, we can understand neoliberalism as the "government of individualization—a form of governance that tasks itself with the production of individuals able to function in a world conceived of as a market, and that are capable of being managed by regulatory economic principles of competition and enterprise."[80] Accordingly, William Davies argues that creating equivalence between subjects is a necessary precondition for the implementation of modalities of market competition.[81] For Davies, neoliberalization "depends precisely on *constructing or imputing certain common institutional or psychological traits, as preconditions of the competitive process*. These serve as principles of equivalence, via which legitimate forms of non-equivalence can be quantified, constructed, represented, and celebrated."[82] Neoliberal subjects are enjoined to see themselves as bundles of self-cultivated skills, which can be traded in an equal labor market; their relationships, as resources to be weighed up to further their self-interested goals in an open field; and their lives, as ventures of ever-expanding personal development restricted by nothing other than their own application and positive psychological motivation.[83] Individuals are asked to develop, grow, and build themselves in order to win at the game of life. Most significantly, the story that is often told here, of the fair competition said to exist between all individuals at all times, pivots upon the assumption that every individual starts from the same place to begin with, with the same opportunities available to all. This component is crucial. Legitimate competition requires an equal field of social relations, and subsequent rankings can carry weight, and thus persuasiveness, only upon this basis. Through this lens, it becomes easy to justify the inequalities we witness in society, such as those observable in well-being on Facebook, by attributing personal responsibility to those who seem to do well, and to those who seem to perpetually lose.

In Facebook's earliest HCI studies, which have been the subject of analysis for the second half of this chapter, similar notions of meritocratic marketized equivalence permeate the discussion surrounding social capital and well-being. Here, there is a sense that the different levels of social support that different users experience on the platform are the result of good or bad personal behavioral decisions. For instance, the loneliness felt by one user as opposed to another can be correlated with the levels of active communication engaged with. The user who is more active on the platform is the more connected, healthier user. In contrast, the user who is more passive, who does not engage with the platform as much, is the lonely, unhealthy one. This appears to be an easy, uncontroversial equation. To live well on the platform, all the user needs to do is cultivate the social resources already at their disposal. Be more active, communicate with your ties, live well. The thought of American sociologist James S. Coleman is a key reference used by Facebook to conceptualize this operative relationship between social capital and well-being.[84] Developing the notion of human capital espoused by Gary Becker and Theodore Schultz in the 1960s, which takes the unique capacities of the human actor as differentials of value in the labor market, Coleman's theory of social capital, as implemented by Facebook, seeks to extend the remit of market rationality to the totality of social relations.[85]

Coleman suggests that social capital is an economically functional concept, attributing value to the potentially productive relations that exist between persons. In this way, Coleman considers social capital in tandem with the concepts of financial, physical, and human capital and the situation of value in money, factors of production, and personal skills, respectively.[86] With his version of social capital, Coleman seeks to "import the economists' principle of rational action for use in the analysis of social systems proper, including but not limited to economic systems, and to do so without discarding social organization in the process. The concept of social capital is a tool to aid in this."[87] For Coleman, and within Facebook's research explicated so far, self-interest thus forms the theoretical basis upon which social organizations can be studied. Users are conceived as detached atoms primarily connected by the availability of social capital resources. Human relationships on Facebook, as has been outlined above, are said to have value according to the perceived benefits they can provide for the individuals involved.

In the world of healthy users, relationships are resources. Friendship, love, sociality, and all the variety of human life online equate with networking. Well-being is a self-interested pursuit. Social support is given only if it can be reciprocated. While Facebook's version is blunt, and not representative, it can reasonably be argued that all theories of social capital provide a poorly instrumental account of the value of human relationships, by leaving little room to view personal connections as anything other than opportunities for personal progression. Moreover, some have suggested that conceptualizing social relations in economic terms forms part of a broader neoliberal project that sees economic rationality being extended to formerly noneconomic social domains and institutions. Sociologists Emanuele Ferragina and Alessandro Arrigoni, for example, argue that "the reduction of social relations to something similar to financial capital" assumes that forms of "social participation are forms of economic activity."[88] Indeed, Foucault's 1978-79 lectures at the Collège de France argue something similar. In these lectures, Foucault describes the rationality of neoliberalism as a generalized attempt to "use the market economy and the typical analyses of the market economy to decipher non-market relationships and phenomena which are not strictly and specifically economic but what we call social phenomena."[89] As such, social capital could justifiably be considered a neoliberalized epistemology, regardless of how it is implemented, by offering marketized concepts to interpret previously un-marketized domains.

These are fair and warranted critiques. However, Facebook's utilization of social capital is particularly neoliberalized even when we leave these broader concerns related to the concept to one side. This is because competing theories of social capital, not to mention several empirical studies, attempt to show that the levels of social support individuals perceive themselves to retain cannot be separated from existing inequalities, which often follow distinctly class-based, gendered, and racialized trajectories. This, in turn, can be closely related to the aforementioned "social determinants of health" framework, which highlights how structural forces delimit how different individuals are able to experience health in different societies at different times. Rather than the differences in social capital being the sole result of personal decisions on Facebook, as we are led to believe in the discourse of active/passive use, we should instead recognize that different users, from different social groups, may experience different levels of social capital on the platform, and thus depreciated well-being, for reasons well beyond their choosing or control.

Pierre Bourdieu, for example, demonstrates how class shapes the access to social capital resources one enjoys within their social context.[90] Bourdieu argues that being born into differently classed social groups opens up different ranges of social possibility for the individuals within them. Those born into material wealth, for instance, perhaps within a social network comprising professional workers, have increased access to potentially productive social contacts when compared to an individual born into poverty. As an example, note how the opportunity for an informal internship within a workplace, wherever that may be, depends upon appropriate recommendations, or a contact already in that place of work. If very few of the social contacts that surround you are in stable employment, with recommendations hard to come by as a result, we can see how this type of opportunity could appear to be very slim for individuals growing up in disadvantaged circumstances.

While this is not to say that the material circumstances one is born into determine the style of life one can live, or the type of work one can engage in, we must acknowledge that social opportunity is not an equal prospect enjoyed on a level playing field. This contrasts with meritocratic discourses, which display a tendency to view those enjoying the trappings of success as inherently deserving of them in some way. Those individuals with high salaries in high-profile jobs have obviously worked harder, done more, and been *better* than those on lower rungs of the salary scale. Their material success is their own doing—congratulations to them. Following this logic, happy, healthy users of Facebook are simply reaping the rewards of their own positive communication choices. The unhappy ones, meanwhile, are just not trying hard enough to follow suit. While these are obviously fairly brusque examples, this thinking undergirds much of the discourse surrounding inequality today, and the ideals of meritocracy are often invoked to justify political inaction on inequality, unemployment, and poverty. When material success and psychological well-being are imagined to be all up to the individual, both the value and the need for either meaningful thought or applicable sociopolitical interventions are negated. Those enjoying material and psychological security, as such, are placated with the idea that it was their own doing, and their own doing alone, that granted them the stable positions they are currently in. Correspondingly, others who find themselves in less lucrative circumstances can be considered to have only themselves to blame.

However, when we acknowledge that social capital, and the opportunities it brings, is in large part *inherited*, and perhaps not solely down to personal choice and behavior, the persuasiveness of these meritocratic ideals begins to dissolve. What Bourdieu's thought encourages us to do is instead draw attention to the way privilege actually operates. It seems that having friends in high places, while a cliché, can in fact be viewed as an operative social dynamic. Overall, we should recognize that social capital does not exist on an equal plane, simply to be grabbed, utilized, and made to work for us all equally. Access to opportunity is structural. So are its inequalities. This is in contrast to Facebook's version of social capital and well-being, which is an inherently individualized prospect.

The false social equality that underpins neoliberal myth-making is demonstrably inaccurate, as Bourdieu and others, like Jo Littler, can show.[91] Yet despite this, such ideas are incredibly procreant, as this present analysis of Facebook's discourse of responsibilized well-being reveals. In appropriating scales of equivalized social capital as its chief measure of well-being, I argue that Facebook is relaying a historicized conceptualization of the self-interested, competitive human subject that perpetuates a hegemonic neoliberal worldview. Adopting this view of social relations limits our ability to imagine well-being as anything other than a personal achievement or failure. We either choose to win the competition of well-being or not. In this way, Facebook's vision obscures the unchosen structural fields that cradle inequalities in social capital and well-being in the present day, which always exist prior to, and alongside, individual decisions of healthy active use. This obfuscation, as I will explore more in the following section, intentional or not, functions as what Foucauldian scholar Tiisala describes as a mode of *topical exclusion*, whereby power works to exclude potential angles of collective interpretation of particular social phenomena.[92] As a result, rather than being simply viewed as forming part of Facebook's PR strategy of healthy use,

Facebook's discourse of well-being actually has real political effects by bringing neoliberal imaginaries of social responsibility into public consciousness, and excluding others. If we are to properly appreciate how social media use is related to operative well-being inequalities, we need to move beyond these constraining analytics and imaginaries and approach the question in new terms.

The Current Political Limits and Future Potential of Social Media Well-Being

Through Facebook's neoliberal lens that we have been examining so far, well-being on the platform is conceptualized chiefly as an outcome of individual decision-making—the choice of active use and the cultivation of social capital it brings. However, as already discussed in the introduction, scholars in several disciplines have shown how negative experiences of well-being—as manifested in anxiety, depression, fatigue, or low self-esteem, for instance—are distinctly relational, involving neurological, hormonal, and behavioral processes interacting with subjective experiences of adverse environmental conditions.[93] Various configurations of gender, race, class, and physical capacity pressure individuals differently in the world, resulting in uneven likelihoods that individuals may experience psychological difficulties throughout their lives.[94] Public health scholar Matt Fisher, for example, shows how living in hostile social environments—where racism, sexism, and ableism are operative, for instance—can be correlated with the increase of stress hormones in the body, leading to increased physical and psychic tension that works to negatively impact feelings of well-being as a result.[95]

However, Facebook studies and speaks to its users as if they exist in a technological vacuum, divorced from these environing social conditions. This is hugely significant. In ignoring the structural factors important to well-being—adequate housing, health, work, income, and structural fairness, for instance—Facebook's vision of individualized well-being is unable to highlight how inequalities in these areas are crucial factors in societal and individual feelings of unwellness, foreclosing both the ability and the subsequent *need* to address such issues from a psychological standpoint. This constitutes an inherently political foreclosure, a mode of *topical exclusion*, that entrenches ideological visions of an atomistic society inhabited by self-contained, and self-reliant, neoliberal agents, split from the social world around them. Whether conscious or not, Facebook's vision of its ideal users and ideal pathways of living well online maintains neoliberal worldviews.

In Facebook's psycho-computational configuration of healthy active use, individual users walk a path to positive well-being simply by making optimal—marketized—choices of healthy living. This resonates with the broader neoliberalization of mental health care in the Global North since the 1980s.[96] In lieu of state-provided mental health welfare, whether because of its actual nonexistence or its de facto ineffectiveness due to limited funding (as in the UK), individuals are tasked with making changes to their lifestyle in order to ameliorate their subjective feelings of negative well-being.[97] This frequently involves suggested changes in diet, exercise routines, sleep patterns, and stress management techniques.[98] We can now add to this list the management of activity and time spent on social media. This means that the individual must avoid "unhealthy" actions as they navigate their way through life (passive social media use, for instance) and adopt "healthy" actions (like active social media use) in order to live well. As Wendy Brown demonstrates, this results in the production of neoliberal subjects of "self-care," whose moral worth is predicated on their "ability provide for their own needs and service their own ambitions."[99]

Yet, by assuming that all individuals are equally disposed to choose healthy lifestyles, and by placing the burden of health solely on individual choices alone, neoliberal conceptualizations of responsibilized well-being, like Facebook's, divert attention away from the wider circumstantial fields that structure the range of choices open to individuals at any given moment in time. For instance, despite what the broader wellness discourse says, people still need spare time in order to exercise, sufficient money to purchase nutritious food, working arrangements that facilitate routine, and dependable screen and sleep patterns. So-called "good" choices are thus prestructured by contingent social, financial, and environmental circumstances. Facebook's vision of self-interested well-being makes it difficult to address these issues by presenting social media well-being as simply a matter of *good active choices*. While the ability to correlate increased passive social media use with increased depression and anxiety is undoubtedly important for clinical treatments, we ought to also recognize that the individual tendency for depression and anxiety is unevenly distributed throughout the social body prior to its manifestation in online contexts. The free and equal choice of well-being online, in other words, is not quite as straightforward as Facebook says. Scholars working in the critical medical humanities, such as Sarah Atkinson, move away from discussing well-being in terms of personal habits and individual failings in favor of a more relational view of well-being that is better able to account for the social and environmental factors involved in human flourishing.[100] Atkinson and colleagues offer a community-based model of well-being that grants a "greater focus on social and collective life."[101] This view focuses on "our relations with the diverse processes and places that hinder or enable us to become well together."[102] Here, living well is not the sole outcome of individual choice, but is dependent on sustaining and supportive community relations.

Elsewhere, Sarah C. White considers well-being as an emergent process, something "that happens in and over time through the dynamic interplay of personal, societal and environmental structures and processes, interacting at a range of scales, in ways that are both reinforcing and in tension."[103] The human subject of well-being is said to be produced through these dynamic processes in a way that complicates the prioritization of personal autonomy and choice. White's view of well-being is instead grounded in "a relational ontology that views relationality as logically prior to individuals, rather than vice versa. It celebrates multiplicity and resists fixity, seeking always to extend possibilities for relationship."[104] In this way, the "subjective, material and relational dimensions of well-being are revealed as co-constitutive."[105]

White's intra-active approach has the potential to challenge Facebook's view of well-being, instead allowing us to examine processes of technological mediation in analytical tension with specific sociopolitical circumstances. For example, rather than simply correlate negative well-being outcomes on social media with poor behavioral choices, we could begin to examine the structural factors that create uneven feelings of well-being in communities as they entwine with the affordances of social media. This type of analytic reorientation works to decenter behaviorist logics and the tired battle between structure and agency, instead allowing the broader sociotechnical issues surrounding social media well-being to come to the fore. In doing so, we become better equipped to fully understand how the technical design of social media platforms, which are undoubtedly designed to extract value from user attention for capitalist gain, may detrimentally impact some groups of users more than others. This would lift the burden of "fixing" social media well-being from the individual user alone, opening up new connections between feelings of digital unwellness and unequal dynamics of power "offline."

When well-being is associated with environing relations and specific times and places "involving the intimate flow of life-courses, inter-generational relations, processes of stability and sustainability," new types of personal interpretation, policy measures, sites of intervention, and collective action that can address these issues become relevant.[106] Facing up to hereditary inequities, prejudice, discrimination, and environmental disparities, for instance, suddenly becomes crucial in attempts to ameliorate human well-being in any given arena. What is more, the variegated psychosocial experiences of negative well-being, once associated with structural, *unchosen* factors, produce common points of political pressure. Rather than the feelings associated with negative well-being—anxiety, depression, and low self-esteem, for instance—resulting from the behavioral and psychic faults of the individual, such feelings become viable entry points to discuss the structural forces that, while in no way determinate of them, are involved in their expression. The force of these ostensibly negative feelings can then be productively turned outward instead of only in.

Refusing the Terms of Engagement

To recall a key theme that runs throughout this book, and as STS scholar Madeleine Akrich argues, technologies can "stabilize, naturalize, depoliticize, and translate" social relations to such an extent that it can often appear as if there were "never any possibility it could have been otherwise" in the world.[107] This chapter has sought to open up these possibilities by exposing the historical scientific contingencies upon which Facebook establishes its visions of ideal healthy use. I have shown how Facebook's recommendations are made through the peculiar blending of evolutionary and neoliberal discourses, and have made a case for why we should do our best to reconsider the matter through new terms. I have revealed the ways in which Facebook seeks to present the engineered sociality observable on the platform as the culmination of rational users acting in alignment with their natural needs. This type of active use, rather than being viewed as the result of a designed user experience intended to gather data for the sake of capitalist profit, is instead singularly presented as the result of rational user choices fulfilling innate, natural, human social needs. This presentation rests upon artificial models of the neoliberal competitive subject and, as such, always exists in a necessary process of construction. Accordingly, Facebook's concurrent appeal to evolutionary human need can be seen as a strategic attempt to naturalize what is an inherently contrived vision of human sociality—a process of attempted stabilization that Langlois and Elmer have examined in terms of "proprietorial enframing."[108] With this in mind, rather than aligning with the fabricated innate needs of users, I have argued that Facebook's psycho-computational configurations of healthy social networking habits are better viewed as expressions of governance that link users to contemporary orders of digital capitalism and historical discourses of neoliberalism.

Facebook's account of well-being responds to the very real criticisms that were being leveled at its services in the mid- to late 2010s. Focusing on the benefits of active healthy use provides reasons for users to continue to interact with the platform, which, in doing so, keeps open profitable channels of datafication for its owners and shareholders to benefit from in the future. However, the broader effects of this apparatus of governance extend far beyond its inceptive strategic, behavioral, economic functions. I have also shown how Facebook's psycho-computational configuration of healthy use makes it very difficult to link any inequalities of social capital, loneliness, and depression observable on Facebook to either the design of the platform or the wider social inequalities experienced in contemporary neoliberal capitalist societies. If, as sociotechnical researchers, we wish to draw attention to these salient factors, we would do well to move beyond the categories and terms provided by social media companies, and the technology industry in general, to conduct our analyses. By taking up hegemonic concepts and forms of measurement, like active and passive use—which are endorsed and repeated by interested technological actors—our epistemological horizons are restricted to predefined terms of engagement, terms that curtail what can be said about certain phenomena and what cannot. On this exact point, Tarleton Gillespie writes: "Solving the problems the industry created on the terms they offer can lead us to overlook the problems we are not being invited to solve, the communities the industry tends to ignore, the solutions that challenge the business models embraced by the industry, and those dilemmas that are in fact not solvable, but are actually meant to be perennially contested."[109] Moreover, following the thought of Sara Ahmed, failing to question the concepts and measures through which we examine social media could risk uncritically accepting the visions of the world that are peddled by their corporate owners. This acceptance is not arbitrary, but is "what blocks other possible worlds" from emerging.[110] To make a horribly banal point, then, the concepts through which we choose to examine the world require our utmost care and attention.

In particular, opening up the location and scale of our analysis to broader terrains that may not immediately, on the surface, seem relevant can widen the scope to include previously marginalized perspectives. It is up to critically minded researchers, acting with whatever agency is still left in the ability to research, write, and speak, to decide what is relevant to study, and how to go about it, rather than simply following readymade interpretations of the topic offered by certain interested groups. In highlighting the contingencies and analytic foreclosures located within Facebook's discourse of healthy active use, I hope to have demonstrated an example of the generative potential of this type of academic activity.

To close, accepting or rejecting Facebook's potion of healthy use remains a personal choice, yet this chapter has argued that we should all at least know its active ingredients before we take a drink. This involves public audiences not simply taking recommendations of the digital good life at face value, but more importantly for researchers to be wary of the analytics we use to assess the value, purpose, and political effects of so-called healthy social media use in the present age. This chapter has shown what insights can be gained if we do not simply take the worlds imagined by social media companies for granted, or accept the concepts through which we are led to understand them. When we subject culturally commonsense visions of well-being to sustained critical scrutiny, we often find that the logics holding them together may not align with our own political sensibilities. This potential disconnect could be the starting point for new ways of thinking about the social, cultural, and technological ties that social media currently bind, opening up new threads for us to loosen for ourselves, and points of pressure to relieve for others as a result.

2 *Neuroliberal Interfaces*

We're going to introduce something which I think will make a considerable difference, which is where our systems see that the teenager is looking at the same content over and over again, and it's content which may not be conducive to their well-being, we will nudge them to look at other content.

NICK CLEGG, president of global affairs at Meta

We know you want to be able to control your experience on social media in a way that works for you and supports your well-being. That's why we've rolled out features that let you manage your time, prevent unwanted interactions and control what type of content and accounts you see. Here are some examples of reminders and nudges that are now live.

META, Health and Well-Being Safety Center

As the quotes above indicate, the types of interventions that Meta deems useful in the struggle for user well-being are saturated with the language of nudge. This chapter will explore the political implications of this discursive alignment, demonstrating how the normative thresholds of nudge and its circumscribed constructions of personhood, choice, and freedom are materially expressed through the wellbeing designs of social media platforms like Facebook. Drawn from the work of American behavioral economists Richard Thaler and

Cass Sunstein, the core idea of nudge states that subtle design decisions can adjust human behavior in particular directions in order to meet positive health outcomes.[1] Examples include arranging school cafeterias in a way that prioritizes nutritious food choices, engraving house flies on public urinals to improve aim and hygiene, opt-in donor schemes that increase benefactor pools, and, indeed, designing social media in a way that fosters "healthy" active communications and self-controlled use. Nudge concerns itself with creating *choice architectures* that are intended to improve human decisions in environmentally constrained situations, using contextual cues to effect intended goals.[2] Here, encouraging "better" choices through design is imbued with an ability to structure a person's journey toward their own personal flourishing, all the while maintaining an impression of free choice and decision.

The types of interventions suggested by social media platforms to encourage healthy use are established in these behaviorist terms. Instagram, Facebook, YouTube, and TikTok, among others, now all nudge users toward certain actions on platforms, in discourse and design, for the sake of their own well-being. Examples include features that allow users to set limits on the time they spend on certain platforms. These are marketed as a form of conscious use. If such limits are met, platforms send users an alert reminding them to take a break. Other features, such as "quiet" modes, enable users to mute push notifications for set periods, creating temporary barriers that seek to support attentive focus elsewhere, away from the distraction of their feeds. On Instagram, comment reply reminders send automated messages to users to think twice about posting potentially offensive comments. Tellingly, this is a move the platform itself describes as "nudging people to take a beat" before they post something incendiary.[3] Relatedly, kindness reminders encourage "thoughtful and respectful" communications when direct messaging other users, using language detection software for the purpose.[4] More generally, users of Facebook are encouraged to cultivate a social network that "inspires" rather than diminishes feelings of positivity, by blocking certain people and types of posts in their feeds or hiding particular keywords in comment sections.[5]

All of this, in and of itself, seems fairly innocuous. Surely a bit of self-control and positive communication on social media is no bad thing? However, as disconnection studies have shown, and as Ana Jorge and colleagues' work explores in particular, such tools in fact contribute to an *ideology of temporal disconnection* that prioritizes individualized time controls on platforms as the path to social media well-being, at the expense of other interventions. Moreover, for other critical scholars, the focus on controlling personal activity and interactions on platforms has also been shown to obscure the rather limited degree of choice actually available to users to disconnect from social media as a whole.[6] Instead, as I and numerous others have argued elsewhere, social media tools of well-being serve to more deeply entwine users with the psychosocial demands of platforms, increasing self-managed activity and thus working to ensure that profitable avenues of capitalist datafication remain open for interested parties.[7] Nevertheless, as evidenced by the quotes above, the increasing availability and promotion of these tools, which nudge users toward active, controlled, and self-curated use, indicate that social media companies are increasingly committed to presenting an image of paternalistic, yet distanced, care toward their users, in the face of the psychological risks their services seemingly pose.[8]

The perceived necessity of such digital wellness tools, and the healthy habits they aim to cultivate, ought to be understood in relation to broader historical concerns surrounding the impact of digital technologies on the well-being of populations and individuals.[9] In particular, these concerns are related to issues surrounding corporate social responsibility, and the extent to which companies have a duty of care for the safe use of their commercial products in marketized, deregulated, neoliberalized societies.[10] Additionally, the bigger ethical issue of designing computational technologies that do not harm users (which is generally accepted as fairly essential) is now supplemented by the demand for technologies that actively seek to improve the well-being of their users, as part of some sort of universalist, teleological moral imperative.[11] Here we may think of frameworks such as "positive computing" that have emerged from human-computer interaction (HCI) studies, which, for example, seek to create consumer technologies that foster aspirational characteristics of "self-awareness, autonomy, resilience, mindfulness, and altruism" in the hearts and minds of their users.[12] These are capitalist designers that care.

Elsewhere, innumerable applications and devices exist that allow users to measure and improve their well-being online and in their day-to-day lives. These are readily available to consumers, offering the ability to track perceived changes in mood over time, sleep patterns, or levels of stress, for example.[13] Other applications provide space for users to practice mindfulness, meditation, or breathing exercises for relaxation, and a vast array are focused on supporting physical activity and user fitness.[14] Again, all of this shouldn't be taken at face value—these are not unproblematic tools that simply help users on a path to the good life. Rebecca Jablonsky, for instance, shows how repeated interactions with commercial meditation applications offer users a promissory veneer of attentive control, obscuring the real ways that their thoughts and behavior are, ironically, being shaped by the technologies of nudge contained within the applications' design—for a directly datafied (economic) purpose.[15] Indeed, the majority of these well-being technologies, as well as the tools tailored toward social media well-being mentioned above, likewise directly intervene in the habits and routines of their users through various nudge interventions that foster continued engagements. These include sending reminders to complete certain tasks, creating engagement scores that track daily use, providing default activity settings, recommending modes of use, and using non-forcible language to encourage change, through simplified "user-friendly" designs. As such, and as seen with the kind of wellness applications highlighted so far, nudge has been enthusiastically taken up by practitioners working in technology companies, by scholars in the related discipline of HCI, and by commercial social media companies to demonstrate how their products can not only be profitable, but can also help improve human decisions and, ultimately, improve human lives.[16]

In the ethically loaded frameworks of nudge, the creation, ideas behind, communication, and dissemination of computational designs and products serve an inherently normative function. This immediately undercuts the tool-views of technology explored in the introduction, which may seek to frame technologies like social media as neutral, empty vessels that only become morally charged when wielded by autonomous users for their own ends. Instead, as design theorist Johan Redström argues, the tool-view of technology is untenable due to the human-made quality of designed objects themselves, which express contingent norms tied to the particular aims of the designer, and the stated usefulness and value of the technology in question.[17] Insofar as "a given thing could always have been designed differently," human-designed objects, environments, systems, arrangements—whatever, and whatever you want to call them, "do not only present and represent a certain point of view that can be contested, they also act as a kind of argument in favour for adopting that particular point of view."[18] These arguments demand a response from users, without necessarily determining their interactions. As such, all design ought to be considered a rhetorical statement, as opposed to a neutral utterance; a persuasive gesture, rather than an impartial intervention.[19]

Accordingly, to distinguish one particular school of design as supremely, or more perniciously, persuasive than all others is fallacious. And as Redström suggests, this is a shaky basis for discursive claims about the uniqueness of persuasive computing, largely associated with B. J. Fogg and popularly encountered in the critiques of the devilishly dark patterns of social media design.[20] While the intention to direct behavior through design may be more or less strong in the consciousness and actions of particular designers and design teams, and the functionality of particular technologies may be more or less open to creative interpretation by users, this variability does not change the core rhetorical operation of something being designed *this way*, rather than *that*. What is more, it is important to recognize that these forms of design persuasion necessarily construct a user that is there to be persuaded—a being imagined to have certain proclivities, levers of motivation, assumed desires, needs, pressure points, capacities, and wants (as examined in some depth in chapter 1). Following Madeleine Akrich, this is usefully framed as a form of technological scripting, which "defines a framework of action together with the actors and the space in which they are supposed to act," as articulated by the design of technologies and their imagined contexts of use.[21]

Thus, when seeking to analyze discourses and designs of social media well-being, which is a key aim of this book, and the normative values they present and promote, other empirical avenues of exploration emerge beyond the obvious digital wellness tools outlined above, which a strong body of existing literature has already productively examined to date.[22] This chapter builds on such research but seeks to draw our attention to the normative functioning of other, less obvious aspects of platforms' nudge *choice architectures*. Drawing once again on the case study of Facebook that ties the empirical chapters of this book together, I will show how Facebook's intention to build and maintain products that are "good for people, and good for society" is not only a discursive argument, but also a material one embedded in the design of Facebook's various technical functions and user interfaces.[23] This chapter will select a single, yet crucial, feature of Facebook's user-interface choice architecture, the Feed, in order to add some empirical specificity to these arguments.

Feed / Power

The Feed occupies the user's home page of Facebook, constituting an algorithmically ranked rolling stream of (sometimes sponsored) content emerging from the user's personal social network. Facebook's Help Center states: "Feed is the constantly updating list of stories in the middle of your home page. Feed includes status updates, photos, videos, links, app activity and likes from people, Pages and groups that you follow on Facebook."[24] Upon its release as the "News Feed" in 2006, some users weren't pleased with the lumping together of their disparate Facebook activities within a singular interface.[25] That change in design was imagined by some scholars as a form of "context-collapse."[26] In the years since, after innumerable iterations and a name change, and despite now being a relatively stable part of Facebook's platform, the Feed has continued to court controversy. Chiefly, this centers on the way the Feed orders and presents information to users. Here we may think of popular arguments about "filter bubbles" and "echo chambers," which suggest that the personalization of content on the Feed creates individual information silos that undermine the formation of shared publics, while simultaneously polarizing political and cultural forms of communication toward extremes. This is often related to the so-called attention economy, whereby outrageous viewpoints, fake news, misinformation, and disinformation (all garnering intense reactions) climb up the Feed for their purveyors and for Facebook to profit from, economically and otherwise.[27] Frequently as a result, the political significance of Facebook's Feed is often presented as contributing to nothing less than the downfall of public political communication, rational debate, and the saliency of Truth (with a capital T). In these controversies, the very grounds upon which liberal democratic forms of government are built and sustained are viewed as under attack.

These critiques, obviously, stem from an ideological commitment to the imagined liberal democratic public sphere and a particular account of how the circulation of information contributes to its proper functioning. However, other forms of critical scholarship have examined the political significance and social controversies of the Feed through alternative conceptual rubrics. For example, Ilana Gershon considers the ranking of information on the Feed through its neoliberal logics, exploring how the public ordering of information rearticulates intimate communication in competitive terms.[28] Other scholars engage with, and invert, Foucault's concept of panoptic discipline to understand the Feed's normative significance.[29] Taina Bucher, for example, argues that having posts prominently placed on others' Feeds is an aspirational aim inculcated in users through the competitive ranking and metrification of content on the interface.[30] Elsewhere, Benjamin Grosser describes the social metrics on the Feed as a "graphoticon[,] . . . a form of self-induced audit . . . where the many watch the metrics of the many."[31] For these authors, rather than an omniscient authority enforcing behavioral norms from a singular vantage point, users observe and assess the behavior of other users in a process of networked self-administration, as set out by the affordances of the interface itself. Interestingly, Facebook and Instagram have recently introduced the ability for users to hide the public visibility of metrics on their posts, which may alter the force of these interpretations. However, and significantly, it remains that users are still privately met with metrics for their own posts whenever they log in to the platform. Thus, Foucauldian concepts of surveillance, by focusing on the feeling of assessment and changes in behavior that panoptic regimes engender, allow us to relate the systems of ordering and measurement found on the Feed (privately constituted or otherwise) to processes of disciplinary power.

This chapter will offer an alternative consideration of the normative functioning of the Feed through slightly different, but related, Foucauldian-inspired analytics of governance. Primarily, the way the Feed offers an argument for healthy active use through its design and accompanying discourses will be understood as a targeting of conduct. Principally, this is because the structuring of nudged choice on the Feed's user interface produces the profitable data-traces necessary for Facebook's capitalist functioning *through*, not in spite of, users' ostensibly free capacity to choose how they interact with the platform. Accordingly, the chosen modes of use that the Feed encourages work upon the thoughts, freedom, actions, and habits of users, shifting behavior in certain directions, proposing subject positions to adopt, to be taken up or resisted, incorporated or withstood, enthusiastically or reluctantly, consciously or not—all the while working in Facebook's economic interests. Through this lens, this chapter will situate the Feed's nudged design as a constituent element of contemporary neuroliberal apparatuses of governance—which seek to influence behavioral decisions through intervening in "both the situations in which decisions are made and the emotional drivers of those decisions."[32] Keep in mind the definition of *neuroliberalism*: "the increasing capacity of states, corporations, and non-governmental organizations to govern through a series of more-than-rational registers of human action (including habits, heuristics, emotions, affects, and social and environmental contexts), and to skilfully fuse behavioural power with liberal notions of freedom."[33] This chapter will position the Feed as a *neuroliberal interface*, seeking to govern its users "through the psychological appropriation of [digital] spaces" that have supposedly been designed in terms of their own well-being interests.[34]

My argument in this chapter will thus expand the concept of neuroliberalism into new empirical terrains, chiefly through an examination of the stated design ethics behind the Feed, as well as a material analysis of the interface itself. Before this, however, it is important to more clearly establish the grounds upon which Facebook imagines itself as an appropriate arbiter of human conduct in the first place. To do this, we must turn to the psychologized discourses of nudge through which Facebook justifies, positions, and actualizes itself as a benevolent provider of services that can satisfy the imagined well-being needs of its users. The following section will examine the core ideas and assumptions behind this positioning, providing some useful theoretical and historical context to the now normal idea that social media companies somehow have the right to construct and structure their users' behaviors in certain directions as opposed to others.

Nudge

The idea of nudge works upon a few core assumptions about human nature. We can identify what these assumptions are by looking at the three primary mechanics of nudging, which target contrasting elements.[35] The first mechanic that seeks to affect behavioral change is the use of defaults in design. These defaults take different forms depending on context. On social media, we may think of the default choice in user interfaces; in governmental settings, how administration forms are designed; or the way various companies word their consumer agreements. In nudge, people encountering these defaults are more likely to stick with the options they suggest, rather than changing them. This is explained through the belief that humans are inherently prone to inertia, choosing the path of least resistance whenever possible in order to preserve their own valuable time and energy. Call it efficient or call it lazy, the idea is that the average human would rather leave things as they are than actively choose to change. Defaults work simply by being defaults. Designers and policymakers working with nudge, known as *choice architects* in Thaler and Sunstein's terminology, are encouraged to take advantage of this inertia to achieve certain goals, well-being-related or otherwise. For example, to encourage "greener" behaviors, one study from environmental psychology suggests that setting renewable sources of energy as the default option for electricity utilities will increase the likelihood that consumers will stick with that option in their choice of energy provider in the future.[36]

Sitting alongside this view of human inertia in nudge is the contrasting characteristic of human impulsivity. Here, humans are said to tend toward shortsighted decision-making, prioritizing immediate gain at the expense of long-term planning. Humans, it seems—to nudge theorists at least—will most likely choose the alluring choice rather than the sensible one. This leads to the second key mechanic of nudge: space for reflection. To encourage greater prudence, choice architects are urged to interrupt the flow of this impulsivity, offering moments of reflection to help people navigate important decisions. We can think of the "cooling-off" periods that are built into various administrative processes as examples of this in action—the consumer's right to cancel certain contracts before a set period, for instance, or timing rules around marriage, such as the UK's requirement that citizens post a twenty-eight-day notice before they can be legally wed. On social media, think of the break in activity that comes when reminding users whenever they have reached a certain time limit on their social media feeds.

Finally, the third major mechanism of nudge uses social norm reinforcements to pressure individuals along corridors of activity in certain environments. If the average individual perceives everyone else to be adopting a similar style of behavior in a particular location, over others, that individual will most likely adopt those behaviors as well, rather than stick out from the norm. The assumption is that human beings tend toward conformity and will most often use the existing behaviors of others as guidelines for their own behaviors in various situations. This is often referred to, not unproblematically, as the *herd mentality*. For example, some economists suggest that simply informing individuals about the energy conservation practices of neighbors can lead to changes in their own consumptive practices as they seek to follow suit.[37] Interestingly, this seems to work both ways: often, those who find out they are using relatively more energy than their neighbors decrease their use, while those who find out they are using less increase their consumption.

Overall, in these nudge frameworks, the time to honor the human as the triumphant utility maximizer is over. *Homo economicus* is gone. Instead, we are presented with a figure of the human whose attempts toward rationality are repeatedly thwarted by their own innate fallibility and lack of self-awareness. American political scientist Herbert Simon was one of the first to systemize this apparent human fallibility into a psychological model of individual decision-making.[38] Simon gives us the term *bounded rationality*, which describes how rather than optimizing every decision, at every moment, in every new situation, humans most often use heuristics (interpretive frameworks) that have served them well enough in the past as the basis of their action. Humans are said to repeatedly use these heuristics in their decision-making, consciously or otherwise, to choose options that *seem* reasonable enough at the time, depending on the situation. This process is termed *satisficing*. The field of new behavioral economics, out of which nudge grew, sought to utilize these insights in the design of the built environment and policy interventions.[39] Practices of nudge were developed to address the aforementioned problems that human irrationality seemingly posed for individuals and society at large.

Psychological frameworks related to nudge have also been developed that likewise advise humans to better understand, and work around, their own rational limits. For example, Daniel Kahneman proposes a vision of the human brain based on "System 1" and "System 2" operations.[40] Basically, System 1 refers to fast, unconscious, and reactive thought and is believed to take up the majority of human thinking and activity. System 2 operations are slower, more considered, logical, and controlled, rarely coming into play in the incessant flow of daily life. For new behavioral economists like Thaler and Sunstein, as well as HCI practitioners, social media designers, and other technologists wielding the tools of nudge to target the well-being of users, the dominance of System 1 over System 2 processes is often referenced to ground design interventions. However, rather than this being a barrier to effective design, choice architects instead seek to use the imagined cognitive sloppiness of the human being to their advantage. Riccardo Rebonato defines the approach of nudge overall as "a set of interventions aimed at overcoming the unavoidable cognitive biases and decisional inadequacies of an individual by exploiting them in such a way as to influence her decisions (in an easily reversible manner) towards choices that she herself would make if she had at her disposal unlimited time and information, and the analytic abilities of a rational decision-maker."[41] Therefore, it is not the ideal of rationality that is the target of critique in nudge, but rather the failing cognitive abilities of the humans tasked to reach it. As Chad Valasek insightfully points out, this maintains the hierarchical positioning of rational System 2 thinking over uncontrolled System 1 operations.[42] For Valasek, this works to entrench historicized, colonial, and racialized binaries of the primitive mind in need of civilized cultivation by higher faculties. This, as we will return to later, is often administered through the dissemination of disciplinary technologies of the self.

Thaler and Sunstein describe the various levels of nudging as "libertarian paternalism"—the attempt to design social environments that "move people in directions that will make their lives better."[43] Crucially, however, all of this is done while still maintaining an impression of free choice. Thaler and Sunstein explicitly draw upon the thought of Milton Friedman—one of the intellectual pillars of neoliberal economic doctrine—to make this claim. They argue that the libertarian aspect of nudge theory is found in the driving notion that people "should be free to do what they like."[44] In this way, Friedman's refrain that individual freedom is constituted in being "free to choose" the direction, character, and quality of one's life reverberates throughout nudge frameworks—raising pertinent links to processes of neoliberalization that I will explore in more depth below.[45] The paternalistic aspect of nudge theory, on the other hand, establishes the idea that it is "legitimate" to "try and influence people's behavior in order to make their lives longer, healthier, and better," comprising "self-conscious efforts, by institutions in the private sector and also by government, to steer people's choices in directions that will improve their lives."[46] As such, nudging is ethically grounded upon the normative notion that the direction of human choice is valid if such an effort is intended for the good of the individuals involved.

Beyond prompting active use on social media, timeouts for mindfulness on well-being applications, constructing consumer choices, improving toilet hygiene, and fostering longer-lasting marriages, nudge theory has found its way into the highest echelons of present-day liberal democratic policymaking. For example, the UK government has a dedicated "Nudge Unit," officially called the Behavioural Insights Team, tasked with researching and proposing UK governmental policies that promote healthy behaviors, while Sunstein himself was an advisor to the Obama administration and design consultant on the Affordable Care Act of 2010.[47] Elsewhere, governments in the Netherlands, Germany, Japan, Canada, Singapore, Guatemala, and Lebanon have likewise employed population-scale nudges in policy domains.[48] Other international organizations—such as the European Commission, UNICEF, the World Bank, the OECD, Europe-Aid, the World Economic Forum, and USAID—have utilized nudge techniques "to address issues as diverse as loan repayments, fertilizer use, HIV/AIDS, and a range of public health and hygiene initiatives."[49] As mentioned in the introduction, during the early days of the COVID-19 pandemic in 2020, the UK government repeatedly, and vaguely, invoked behavioral economic science to publicly justify regulations that variously tightened or loosened lockdown measures, nudging the population toward practices of social distancing, hand washing, and self-isolation.[50]

However, while nudge theory can be shown to have infiltrated the decidedly neoliberalized institutions mentioned above, it cannot be neatly, and simply, subsumed within the neoliberal frame. First, as detailed at length in chapter 1, whereas neoliberal doctrines aim at the ostensibly rational human subject—a being who is motivated explicitly by their own self-interest, and fully able to intuit and act upon this rationality through intelligent, conscious action—nudge theory instead paints a picture of human psychology and behavior that tends toward irrationality and error. Secondly, the asocial, atomistic neoliberal agent, divorced from the environing world around them, is replaced by an intrinsically social, relational subject, influenced by the makeup of their lived world and the actions of others around them. Thus, if the finely isolated figure of *Homo economicus* reigns supreme in neoliberal political visions, it is the fallible human subject, dependent on social and contextual cues, that populates the neuroliberal world of nudge. Shortsighted, lazy, greedy, easily diverted—the nudge-able human, for Thaler and Sunstein, is more like the socially popular, yet indelibly stupid, figure of Homer Simpson—rather than the idealized Economic Man of old. Humans, so it goes, flail around in a sea of their own ineptitude, making bad decisions, ruining their health, ruining their environments, and, ultimately, ruining themselves.

The ways in which social media companies like Facebook utilize nudge to positively influence the well-being activities of their users, therefore, represent a wrinkle in the discourse of healthy active use examined so far in this book. Chapter 1 demonstrated how Facebook configures its ideal healthy users through appeals to knowledge drawn from the psy-disciplines. Facebook paints a picture of its users as naturally disposed to actively connect with others on the platform for the sake of improving their own private stocks of social capital and well-being. The argument is that actively using Facebook is rational insofar as it maintains the ties of social support necessary for evolutionary human flourishing. Users connect with others to get that hit of sociality they crave, from deep down in the recesses of their internal psyches. Acting upon innate desires through social networking on Facebook should result in improved personal well-being for users, insofar as it allows them to fulfill their species-being as rational human creatures. However, as already indicated, something is awry here. If, indeed, users were naturally compelled to interact with the platform in a healthy manner, why would Facebook need to design tools that nudge users toward these types of active interactions in the first place?

Neuroliberalism

The fundamental shift in how new behavioral economics understands human psychology (and by extension the politicians, app developers, HCI practitioners, and social media companies like Facebook who take up the field's suggestions) have prompted scholars to develop new conceptual rubrics able to track its subsequent effects. Chiefly, the term *neuroliberalism* delineates a transition from a style of incentivizing behavioral change found in classic neoliberal regimes to the type of contextual alterations found in the choice architectures of nudge introduced above. The subtle shift from *neo* to *neuroliberalism*, however, is not one of negation or supplantment. Rather, the term indicates a persistent relationship between the former and the latter that demands sustained critical attention. Neu-roliberal designs of nudge, in other words, are equally as political as the economic rationalities of neoliberalism, despite attempts to couch its import in terms of objective human (ir)rationality, individ-ual freedom, and population-scale well-being.

It is important to note that the term *neoliberalism* is itself unsta-ble, referring at once to general practices of financialization and economization, while also being a specific historical reaction to Keynesian macroeconomics; establishing itself through both the safeguarding of individual freedoms and population-scale behavio-ral management policies; and proceeding simultaneously through deregulation and intense market fiscal interventions. Accordingly, as Wendy Brown writes, neoliberalism "is globally ubiquitous, yet disu-nified and non-identical with itself in space and over time."[51] In re-sponse to this "loose and shifting" milieu, rather than signifying a radical departure from neoliberalism, Mark Whitehead suggests that neuroliberalism is best "thought of as a micro-economic project that works in harmony with the macro-economics of neoliberalism."[52]

In neuroliberalism the focus on individual habits as the key mo-tor of change represents a form of *topical exclusion*, whereby atten-tion is diverted to particular ways of assessing certain public political issues and how to address them, at the expense of others. Specifi-cally, through the neuroliberal lens, the recent historical failures of neoliberal policy and economics—the 2008 financial crash and the subsequent Great Recession, rising inequalities within and between nation-states, global debt, failures to do with climate collapse, and so on—boil down to individuals acting irrationally and making bad de-cisions within those systems, rather than the structural determi-nants, policy decisions, market relations, or labor arrangements that constitute those systems themselves. Simply put, the systemic failures witnessable within these marketized neoliberalized contexts are said to be the result of individuals not acting as they were expected to, or as they "rationally" should have done. First, individual human greed is to blame for these failures—of the bankers, mortgage lenders, those unable to live within their means. Or second, the ineptitude of citizen decision-making is to blame, with people making poor investments and poor decisions. Through this rubric, it is acting rashly—an aggregated failure of individuals to think "slow" or think long-term—that causes cyclical financial, political, and environmental crises, *not* the political, economic, and cultural historical conditions that facilitate and support their emergence and continuation. Behaviors are at fault, not systems.

As Whitehead summarizes, "neuroliberalism reflects a set of responses to neoliberalism that sees economic crisis not as a product of the market system, but behavioural failings within it (it is akin to correcting for human market failures rather than questioning the overall logics of the market system itself)."[53] It follows that to stop market failures happening again, rather than make any radical changes to the economic system within which they reside—perhaps to make it fairer, more equitable, through stronger regulation or wealth redistribution—it is instead on the individual, and the individual alone, to be better, do better, think better, and act better within the status quo. To safeguard against future calamities, that is, nothing needs to change but *you*. This prioritization of behavioral change, and its political effects, has obvious and immediate parallels with the current discourses and designs of self-controlled, active, healthy social media use promoted by companies like Facebook (as explored at length in chapter 1). Moreover, these responsibilized recommendations crop up in solutions to other pressing present-day issues, for example as found in discourses of climate change (bamboo straws, anyone?), obesity (such as the UK government slogan "Eat well, move more, live longer"), and gambling (on which the industry advises: "When the fun stops, stop").[54] To reiterate a core argument of this book, the ways in which we conceptualize, and problematize, healthy ideals of human cognition and behavior, whether in relation to social media or to other societal-scale issues, represent a distinctly political task. Models of healthy behavior and theories of change circulate economies of responsibility and blame, setting particular courses of action as just and appropriate, and, indeed, configuring the very nature of human organization and individual being to be found therein.

In support of this, Gerd Gigerenzer argues that blaming "societal problems exclusively on the individual mind" is a serious miscalculation, not just because it lets institutions, political infrastructures, and economic relations off the hook, but because it forecloses the possibility that other behavioral interventions, such as education, could be equally important drivers of social change.[55] Rather than simply materializing a good decision on people's behalf, Gigerenzer instead suggests that "the true alternative to nudging is education: making children and adults risk savvy. That encompasses statistical thinking and heuristic thinking, and judgments about the limits and possibilities of both approaches."[56] Although Gigerenzer still implicitly endorses rationality as something universally worth striving for, not questioning the colonial epistemological conditions within which rationality emerged as a human ideal, and although he still constructs individuals as somewhat responsibilized risk assessors of their own lives, his argument can still reveal that nudge is a particularly curtailed, and historically contingent, expression of human action.[57] Specifically, nudge leaves little room for human decision before or beyond the point of action itself. If you want people to think more long term, think slower, and so on, Gigerenzer asks, why wouldn't you try to teach and persuade them that it is necessary to do so? Perhaps the reticence of nudge in this regard has something to do with the open-ended, often surprising, and generative nature of learning, which every educator and student knows well. It is hard to predict what outcomes, futures, or realities education can help individuals and groups toward, or what will grow from it. Learning can be structured, but set outcomes cannot be assured. Maybe, once furnished with relevant viewpoints, from many relevant voices, people may not wish to follow the prescriptions of healthy use laid out in current discourses and designs of social media well-being. Social media choice architects are perhaps either scared of this possibility or believe so strongly in the correctness of their convictions that they are willing to foreclose the chance for other outcomes to emerge. The choices on offer in nudge, therefore, are perhaps not as free as we are led to believe.

Regardless of your feelings toward education, or the value (or reality) of human rationality writ large, a core paradox remains at the heart of nudge: If all humans are fallible and inevitably make *poor* decisions, why would we expect choice architects (who are also human) to be able to make *good* ones on their behalf? As Gigerenzer writes, "on the one hand, experts are said to be subject to the same cognitive biases as ordinary people; on the other hand, they are supposed to be rational and discern what people really want or need."[58] Rather than suggest we dwell on this, neuroliberal nudge infrastructures instead emphasize our own imperfection, while encouraging us to simply trust choice architects not only to know better, but to implement materialized strategies that allow us to be the best possible version of ourselves through their activation. Now I will turn to these entangled and related issues of trust, responsibility, and choice, as well as the contradictions apparent within them, that are at stake in recent discourses and designs of better, healthier user interfaces emerging from HCI studies and put to work by capitalist companies like Facebook.

Interface, Action, Power

As highlighted at the start of this chapter, there is no getting around the fact that all design is normative through its arrangement of interaction. Whatever has been designed one way could always have been designed another way. HCI practitioners Christoph Schneider, Markus Weinmann, and Jan vom Brocke suggest that this becomes especially clear in the design of user interfaces.[59] "As in offline environments," the authors write, "online environments offer no neutral way to present choices. Any user interface . . . can thus be viewed as a digital choice environment."[60] The authors note that "digital nudges influence decisions at the point and moment of decision making" and, in particular, work "by either modifying what is presented—the content of a choice—or how it is presented—the visualization of a choice."[61] The example of the mobile payment app Square, found in various online stores, cafés, and restaurants, is an apt illustration. This interface presents a tipping option by default, and customers must choose "no tipping" if they prefer to skip a gratuity.[62] Using the language of nudge introduced above, such a design feature seemingly plays on both the "inertia" and the "herd mentality" of customers, who would most likely stick with tipping rather than actively choose an alternative option. While this digital nudge has an explicitly monetary function, other examples demonstrate how the designs of various user interfaces have been modified to encourage behavior beyond simple financial incentives.

For example, industrial economists Johan Egebark and Mathias Ekström sought to reduce waste paper in offices.[63] Through a simple experiment, they found that changing the default printer option to double-sided print resulted in a 15 percent reduction of paper consumption overall. Elsewhere, James Turland and colleagues hoped to increase the security of Android users' wireless network connections.[64] To do this, they reordered the presentation of available networks by placing the most secure options at the top, while using color coding to label each network's respective security. In domains that target "healthy" habits, Min Kyung Lee, Sara Kiesler, and Jodi Forlizzi experimented with ways to encourage users to choose more nutritious snack choices on a food ordering website.[65] They found that positioning less nutritious "junk" food on separate pages, after "healthier" foods had been presented, resulted in users more likely choosing the latter over the former. Finally, we can recall the various examples of well-being nudges found on social media already presented in this book—such as those that encourage users to take regular breaks from scrolling, or reminders to actively reach out to "close ties" through direct messaging.

Many of these types of morally loaded design interventions are at the heart of recent developments in positive computing, as discussed in the first part of this chapter. However, while it is hard to argue against the inculcation of greener office practices, or more secure wireless networks, encouraging the kind of social media well-being habits targeted in the final examples puts us on more tenuous grounds. If, as discussed in the introduction and chapter 1, human wellness is a culturally relative discursive formation tied to the time and place of its articulation, what makes the choice architects of HCI best able to determine what wellness actually constitutes, for whom, and how? Moreover, following Gigerenzer, why would we assume that choice architects are immune to the inherent human fallibility that their designs are intended to correct?

It is always the case that designing for well-being pins down fluid values into a stable material shape. When a designer—acting from somewhere, at some time—targets human well-being through the affordances of a technical artifact, their vision becomes something tangible for future users—acting elsewhere, at different times—to respond to. Although what well-being means for this designer could well change over time, reflective of its mutability as a concept, the user of the designed technology is offered no such chance to change. Artifacts are more obdurate, relaying the same values over again, becoming freshly operative at each moment of user interaction. Accordingly, recalling the concept of mediation introduced earlier in this book, Latour describes the inscription of such moralized pro-grams of action in material forms as a form of technical *delegation*, or "congealed labour."[66] The redesigns, updates, and new features that modify particular interfaces repeat this process, strangely stabilizing past images of user well-being through its very iteration.

Because of this, the interface, for the philosopher of design Branden Hookway, "determines the human relation to technology and delimits the boundaries that define human and machine."[67] In this foundational, relational process, "the interface," Hookway con-tinues, "constitutes the gateway through which the reservoir of hu-man agency and experience is situated with respect to all that stands outside of it, whether technological, material, social, economic, or political."[68] In the digital well-being nudge frameworks introduced above, this means configuring users as fallible subjects unable to ac-count for the limits of their own decision-making, necessarily requir-ing a helping hand toward optimal states of wellness through various interventions. As users do not know what is good for them, the argu-ment goes, the choice architect can legitimately intervene on their behalf. Norms are operationalized, beliefs are concretized, and users are forced to negotiate, and choose between, actions that are imag-ined to be beneficial for them. All the while, the individual user has little, if any, input into what these actions actually look like. In repur-posing the same justifications encountered in neuroliberal regimes of governance—chiefly by assuming what the user *is* and what needs correcting for them, and by limiting user choice to a few options of action upon this basis—we can explicitly discern the implicit politics that digital nudge architectures circulate.

More than this, however, we should understand the interface as a relational boundary through which its human users become con-fronted with what they are imagined to be, how they are imagined to act, and what they are imagined to want. These assumptions preempt and configure each user's expected interactions with the interface. It is through their actual interactions with the interface that they *become* what is expected. This reflexive process of user-becoming is something that Benjamin Bratton has explored in great depth, with Florian Hadler and Joachim Haupt likewise drawing attention to interfaces as "active agents" in the production of user-subjects.[69] Similarly, Software Studies scholars Florian Cramer and Matthew Fuller identify the way user interfaces arrange choice to "impose and enhance particular workflows, thought modes, and modes of interaction upon or in combination with human users."[70]

In this way, then, the interface organizes networks of action in the Latourian sense—the world of delegation and congealed labor—but also represents what Foucault would explore as the enmeshed targeting of actions *upon* actions—the micropolitics of power that produces exacting human subjects through the conduct of conduct. In other words, the user interface, by inescapably nudging users toward restricted modes of action, *scripts* both micro- and macro-relations of sociotechnical existence, entrenching particular visions of the human being and optimal human functioning, while producing practicing users of a particular style in the process.[71] As we will see with the case of Facebook's Feed below, a whole gamut of conditioning forces can thus come into view when we examine the discourses and designs that accompany social media interfaces, which are supposedly built with the well-being interests of users in mind. Who designed the interface in question? For what ends? How are its users *meant* to relate to the interface? And what does this desired relation reveal?

Facebook's Feed as a Neuroliberal Interface

I argue that the type of wellness scripting encountered on commercial social media user interfaces such as Facebook's Feed should be considered as neuroliberal in quality and effect. This section will show how the Feed governs its users "through the psychological appropriation of spaces," working to set certain styles of user interaction as both more desirable and more possible than others, for particular economic ends.[72] Moreover, by both discursively and technically ordering what it means to be a healthy user at the moment of interaction and beyond, considering the Feed as a *neuroliberal interface* can offer further insights into present-day psycho-computational complexes introduced earlier in this book. Specifically, by aligning the business interests of Facebook as a data platform with the well-being interests of users themselves, determining what ideal, healthy use of the Feed looks like, and the subsequent building of these ideas into the design of the user interface itself, is a nexus point of economic generativity and contemporary governance.

As outlined in the first part of this chapter, this analytic restriction to Facebook's Feed is empirically necessary because Facebook is a complex technological apparatus that affords multitudinous modes of user interaction. For example, alongside interacting with posts on the Feed, users can privately message other users through the Messenger application, scroll through the Timeline, follow Pages, buy and sell products on the Marketplace, access videos through the Watch application, create charity fundraisers, or browse local events on Community groups (among other activities). To validate the methodological style of script analysis that has grounded the approach of this book so far, it is important to first acknowledge the heterogeneity of Facebook's component parts, and then treat the Feed as a singularly scripted user interface that exists in relation to others on the platform as a whole. In taking this approach, I aim to offer a small, but hopefully significant, empirical contribution to the understanding of Facebook's wider nudge architectures for others to develop in the future. Moreover, despite this empirical specificity, it follows that every social media user interface, by contingently structuring choice through their design, can usefully be considered through the lens of nudge. As such, the critiques that follow, which draw out the economic and political effects of this operation, can likewise be applied to other, similarly commercial, social media—all of which necessarily construct and target the behavioral change of their users through digital infrastructures.

The News Feed, as Feed was called until early 2022, was introduced to Facebook users on September 5, 2006. At the time, an official Facebook blog post introduced the new feature to users as such: "News Feed appears on each user's home page as a constantly updating list of news stories about their friends. It is a news aggregator that reports on activity in a user's social network and highlights relevant information about people, activities they have been involved in and other information they have chosen to share. News Feed is personalized to each user and is only viewable by that person."[73] The introduction of the News Feed gave users a more comprehensive overview of activity that occurred within their social networks. Whereas before, users would have to visit specific profiles to view the activity of friends on Facebook, the News Feed automatically presented all the activity that occurred in their social network in a personalized stream of content on the home page. Whenever a user friended another user, for instance, joined a group, or changed their profile picture on Facebook, such activity would now be displayed on the News Feeds of others in their social network, accompanied by a timestamp of it happening.

The activity that appeared on the News Feed was described in the very first blog post that announced its release as the "headlines" of each user's social network. This discursively and materially characterized the social networking activity of Facebook users as *newsworthy* events. Ruchi Sanghvi, a software engineer at Facebook and the author of the blog post that introduced the News Feed to users at the time, makes this notion explicit: "News Feed highlights what's happening in your social circles on Facebook. It updates a personalized list of news stories throughout the day, so you'll know when Mark adds Britney Spears to his Favorites or when your crush is single again. Now, whenever you log in, you'll get the latest headlines generated by the activity of your friends and social groups."[74] The News Feed was thus originally scripted as a space where the lives of users (as represented on Facebook) constitute news to be shared and accessed by others within their social network.

Not long after its release, Facebook also included privacy settings that allowed users "granular control" over which of their activity shows up on the News Feeds of others, as well as controls that can block others' information appearing on their own.[75] This granular control by the user of who gets to see what on the Feed has persisted as a stable feature to the present day. For example, such privacy controls now include the ability of users to select people and Pages they want to prioritize on the Feed ("managing favorites"), and the ability to unfollow, hide, or snooze posts from others. Users are encouraged to actively curate what comes up on their Feeds and which of their activity is seen by others—something Taina Bucher refers to as administering a disciplinary regime of visibility, as explored earlier in this chapter.[76] This style of active curation is further levied by the Publisher feature, which asks users a leading question every time they navigate to their Feed: "What's on your mind, [user name]?" Prominently placed at the top of the interface, users are encouraged to respond in a variety of ways, by posting a photo or video, for example, "tagging" a friend, "checking-in" at a specific location, or sharing a "feeling." This question prompts a decision: Do I answer? If so, how? Do I ignore it? Why? The question to share "what's on your mind," then, generates further open-ended interaction with the Feed, directly inviting a personalized response by addressing users with their profile name. The naming of users is something that Theresa Sauter has shown to be a core process through which Facebook users form intimate habits of self-expression on the platform.[77] While the invitation to curate privacy settings and share on the Feed involves some degree of user decision, that this activity already counts as good activity, and "headline" activity at that, has been materially constrained through the programmatic configuration of the Feed *prior* to those decisions even being considered or acted upon. This binds the user to a restricted material discursive configuration of activity as a result—is this post newsworthy? Is it not? This, it is plain to see, is a rather limited choice.

Ranking

Since 2018, Meta has offered a new interpretation of the Feed for its users to adopt. Chiefly, the Feed has been charged with the task of "bringing people closer together."[78] According to Meta's Facebook blog series *News Feed FYI*, the Feed's "top priority" is "keeping you [the user] connected to the people, places, and things you want to be connected to—starting with the people you are friends with on Facebook."[79] As outlined in chapter 1, Facebook validates its claims about what people want to be connected to through its studies on user well-being. That is, users are said to be motivated to engage in active social networking to fulfill a natural desire for social belonging and rational desire to accrue social capital. In this framework, increased connection to loved ones on the Feed is imagined to be what users *want*, specifically by allowing users to maintain the social ties necessary for their well-being.

According to information found across this nebulous network of *News Feed FYI* blogs, *ranking* is the collective name for the series of machine learning algorithms that order posts on the Feed. This algorithmic process sorts through all the content that could appear on each user's Feed and places posts that it predicts the user is most likely to interact with at the top of it.[80] Here, a post is deemed "relevant" if it is predicted to prompt user interaction with it. This primary purpose of ranking was explicated in the blog post that detailed its mission change for the Feed in 2018. Ranking, this blog states, has been designed to "prioritize posts that spark conversations and meaningful interactions between people. To do this, we will predict which posts you might want to interact with your friends about, and show these posts higher in Feed. These are posts that inspire back-and-forth discussion in the comments and posts that you might want to share and react to."[81] Prioritizing relevant content in this way is the default setting of the Feed. Although the Feed does have one other available setting that shows posts in chronological order, the Feed will always revert to its default over time. As we've seen, setting defaults in the design of user interfaces makes certain types of interaction with those user interfaces more likely than others over time. As such, the ranking algorithm can be seen to prompt active user interactions through how it displays personalized content on the Feed.

Across the *News Feed FYI* blogs, Facebook makes repeated gestures toward its own research into well-being to justify the design of the Feed. For example, in a quote found within this series, Mark Zuckerberg explicitly states that the aim to spark interactions between users on the Feed is "based on" Facebook's "own research with leading experts," such as Facebook's own researchers Burke and Kraut, whose work was discussed in chapter 1.[82] Here, we can explicitly see how Facebook publicly justifies the Feed's enticing user interface through an appeal to its own research on social capital and group dynamics.[83]

Facebook has published a series of principles termed the *News Feed Values* that establish these efforts to foster close tie connection in more detail.[84] Along with the commitment to prioritizing posts that prompt active communications between family and friends on the Feed, Facebook claims the Feed should also be informative, entertaining, open to diverse ideas, based on authentic communication, under user control, and under constant iteration.[85] Within Facebook's discourse of well-being, therefore, the notion that Feed should function as a space of active communication can be related to the perceived value of digital social bonds, whereby shared positive experiences on Facebook purportedly provide a sense of evolutionary belonging that strengthens social networks. Here, the Feed is scripted as a resource that can provide support, community, and knowledge resources that can improve the flows of functional social capital for users to benefit from in the future. Elsewhere in Facebook's archive of blogs, Zuckerberg claims that this type of active engagement and high levels of user interaction with content on the Feed constitutes "time well spent."[86] Recalling the findings of chapter 1, by determining what *living well* looks like on Facebook, we can see how Facebook and its representatives are projecting a vision of what the Feed's ideal user is and the type of interactions they should aim to cultivate.[87]

Likes and Navigability

Elsewhere on the Feed, the variable design of the like button on posts in different linguistic regions across the globe can be characterized as a visual cue nudge—understood as the visual positioning of certain features in different environments in order to influence individuals' likelihood of interaction with them. On English-language versions of Facebook, for instance, the like button is positioned on the left of posts. This positioning mirrors the way English-reading users would have learned to approach texts from a young age. Correspondingly, Arabic-language versions of Facebook have the like button positioned on the right, likewise responding to the way Arabic is read from right to left. Such variations in the design of the like button suggest that likes are designed to be the first thing that users see when they view a post.

This designed prominence of the like button is justified by Facebook in the same terms of low-cost healthy relationship maintenance discussed in chapter 1. Leah Pearlman, for example, one of Facebook's former employees credited with the development of the like button in 2009, claims the feature was first intended to grant users the ability to quickly show support of a post without having to go to the effort of writing a comment.[88] This thinking remains intact to the present day—for example, the help section of Facebook suggests that "clicking like below a post on Facebook is a way to let people know that you enjoy it without leaving a comment."[89] This view resonates with Facebook's public conceptualization of the like button as an efficient way for users to engage in forms of social grooming, while simultaneously providing quantifiable metrics of user engagement that provide the basis of the "like economy," as examined by Carolin Gerlitz and Anne Helmond.[90]

Finally, in another post of *News Feed FYI*, Facebook's UX specialists state that the comments feature on posts on the Feed have been iteratively designed to foster active communications.[91] The post outlines how the "readability" of posts has been emphasized in order to prompt user interactions and encourage "better conversations" on the Feed. These changes include increased color contrasts, making typography easier to distinguish; updated, larger like, comment, and share icons on posts; and more visible profile picture icons to show more clearly who's involved in the discussions taking place in the comments section. Furthermore, each user's ability to directly reply to comments in a post has been said to be enhanced and made more accessible through clearer fonts and color contrasts. These types of modifications are intended to make the Feed easier to "navigate," and aim to "help people have more lively and expressive conversations on Facebook."[92] This attempt to encourage "lively" conversations, read alongside Facebook's broader stated intentions to "spark" engagement on the Feed, forms part of the discursive pattern that posits the access to one-to-one conversation as a core component of ideal Feed usership. Thus, the way posts are both spoken about and designed can be seen to shape user choice along certain activity corridors as opposed to others. Whether or not users follow these pathways is another matter. It remains that the signposts have been thoroughly set.

The economic incentives of increasing user engagements on social media through nudging have been well documented, and it is clear to see how increasing interactions on the Feed can, and should, be understood as an extractive relation of capitalist power.[93] That is, more interactions create more data and greater profits. Moreover, others have similarly described how these incentives are built into social media's algorithmic designs, channeling user affect and behavior down particular pathways of interaction for economic gain.[94] Yet when considered alongside the neuro/neoliberal discourses explored at length above, the way Facebook justifies these design decisions in terms of the well-being interests of users reveals an even deeper political function. That is, Facebook's contingent, particular, and profitable organization of human activity on the platform is presented as something that is *beneficial* to users and, indeed, the world at large. The way Facebook constructs users of a particular style, and subsequently governs them as such through normative designs, recalls the liberal paternalistic interventions outlined above. More precisely, nudging Facebook's Feed users toward active interventions is presented as being "good" for them, and the future well-being gains they are said to receive through active use validates the way the ranking algorithm is designed to extract value from their activity as a result. Facebook's discursive and material constructs of well-being therefore function by allowing Facebook to explain and justify its design decisions on a discursive ground far removed from its economic purpose as a data platform.

At this juncture, it is possible to show that the discursive formation of Facebook's ideal natural user, as outlined in chapter 1, is reciprocated, although not perfectly, in the stated design values and materiality of the Feed. The good user of self-interested active connection constitutes the target of algorithmic prediction on the Feed, and its neuroliberal qualities are evident in how the Feed's user interface structures choice, and prompts likely interactions, upon this basis. However, the various nudges outlined above beg a serious question, posed earlier in this chapter, that remains unanswered: If users are naturally predisposed to engage in social connection on the Feed, why do they need to be nudged to do so?

Alternative Transparencies

As I have argued throughout this book, Facebook individualizes user behavior as the sole cause of, and solution to, any well-being issues they may face online. This mobilizes neoliberal discourses of responsibilization and thus serves a decidedly political function. However, this chapter adds nuance to this insight by revealing how the supposed empowerment of users to choose healthy behaviors on the platform is, in fact, undermined by the choice architectures of its user interfaces. Consequently, the way that users are nudged to act in a rational, healthy manner on Facebook discloses a distrust in their ability to do so on their own accord. While repeatedly presented as a natural extension of human sociality, therefore, this in fact shows that the framework of self-interested social networking activity erected in Facebook's discourse of ideal use actually requires careful construction, repeated administration, and constant iteration. In this way, the forms of active repetitious communication that Facebook presents as the key to the digital good life online may not be quite as natural or, indeed, as inevitable as Facebook insists. This designed distrust reflects a core dilemma at the heart of neoliberalism that the historical shift toward *neuro*liberalism seeks to address. While this has so far largely been studied in policy domains, this chapter can demonstrate how commercialized user interfaces of social media also serve as a key site of contemporary neuroliberal governance, thus expanding the efficacy of the concept onto new empirical terrains.

Healthy use creates data, a commodity that, in turn, creates healthy profits. However, much like what we saw in chapter 1, Facebook's public messaging seeks to shape how we interpret this salient economic fact. Rather than its encouragements toward active use being viewed as a means to cultivate more engagements, and thus extract more surplus value from its users, Facebook instead justifies its nudges toward active use in terms of improving user well-being. This is itself justified on the basis of its own psychological research and its vision of user/human nature, forming a secure, readymade interpretive paradigm through which we are led to assess its services. This is a classic obfuscating strategy of corporate transparency: ask these questions, on these terms. In response, rather than simply follow these readymade interpretations, and the salient and widespread issues it *topically excludes*, the role of critical researchers is to be alternatively transparent about the psychological, political, and economic effects produced by social media in various spheres of life. That is, instead of taking Facebook's nudges at face value, as simple efforts to improve well-being on the platform, perhaps we should instead view the designs of ideal use as part of a political technology of power that actually seeks to produce governable and economically valuable users. This alternative form of transparency allows researchers to prioritize the positionality of everyday users of Facebook in their research, rather than the corporate interests involved in their administration.

This chapter has shown how social media user interfaces, such as the Feed, construct and target user needs and capacities through designed nudges, while users, in turn, produce themselves in this image through their ostensibly agentic interactions with them. With this insight, however, I do not seek to invoke either determinist or social constructivist thought. Rather, recalling the conceptual challenge of this book, I hope to have highlighted the productive political effects of the Feed in the way it prompts users toward the "acquisition of disciplines or habits"—far beyond the liberal democratic criticisms concerning filter bubbles, echo chambers, misinformation, and self-control introduced above.[95] The political effects of social media user interfaces, consequently, are to be found in the generation of patterns of interactive behavior, which help ensure the continued proliferation of economically productive, and governable, social relations. Rather than claiming that users of Facebook's Feed can utilize its communication features in any way they wish, or simply parrot Facebook's own psychologized appeals to the benefits of active use, I have offered the reader alternative theoretical heuristics through which they can understand the significance of Facebook's contemporary well-being interventions.

Any habitual engagement with the Feed necessarily entails a negotiation with the particular social human history, ideal modes of self-interested communication, and programmatic accounts that Facebook imparts through its discourses and designs of well-being. While the outcomes of user negotiations with the platform are different depending on user circumstance and location, it is not enough to simply point toward such variations and claim that Facebook is a neutral arbiter of the forms of life enacted upon it as a result. Habitual conduct on the platform, while chosen, always happens through an asymmetric interface relation. Therefore, while ostensibly targeting singularly healthy human behaviors on the Feed, I have instead drawn attention to what Alexander Galloway usefully terms *interface effects*, demonstrating how local user interactions have implications far beyond the discretized agents and their particular worlds.[96] The Feed interface, that is, "performs a shaping" of how we understand user/machine relations, how we can imagine human nature and innate psychological capacities, what we deem to be appropriate paternalistic interventions, and who has the right to administer the contemporary digital good life.[97]

Do we trust Facebook's designers to nudge us in directions that are supposedly good for our well-being? How do we feel about companies couching their operations in terms of our own flourishing? And should we resist such a thorough imbrication of social well-being with the extractive economic operations of capitalist platforms? These are open questions with no simple answers. But by highlighting the ways in which Facebook's neuroliberal visions of the good life function within the governance of user well-being, and how these visions are related to arbitrary, very particular, very political accounts of human nature, I hope to have at least established the necessity of their asking.

It remains to be seen, however, in what ways users themselves are actually reacting to the technical nudging of the Feed environment in their daily lives. Do users recognize their Feed activity in the terms of healthy active communication that Facebook provides? If not, how do they understand it? And how is this imagined to impact their well-being? The following chapter will present the findings of a qualitative interview study designed to answer these questions. I will present findings from interviews conducted with users as they scrolled down the Feed and explore the character, and political implications, of users inhabiting an algorithmic environment whereby their relationships and social networking activities are transformed into news, and ranked according to the likelihood of interaction by others on the platform. In other words, chapter 3 will examine what kind of digital good life users imagine to be possible within the extractive Feed environment, when Facebook has very strong ideas on the matter itself.

3 *Scrolling Guilt, Shame, and Blame*

Fundamentally, I dislike Facebook. I would probably go so far as saying I actually hate it. But that doesn't stop me going on it every single day.

FARAH

I know it is really addictive. The Facebook guys know this. They do everything they can to keep you on there. But I also do feel like it's quite lazy to just be like "Oh, well, it's not my fault, I'm just addicted." Because it's kind of like obese people saying that it's McDonald's' fault for them eating too many McDonald's. So, I definitely think a tiny portion of the fault is with Facebook, but they're only so successful because of users being on it.

AVA

So far, this book has established how current recommendations of active social media well-being construct ideal healthy users in discourse and design. This figure, however, is strangely split insofar as it assumes contrasting subject positions at different points in its scripting. On the one hand, we are told that active communications on social media constitute an expression of each user's innate rational psychology, a naturally occurring phenomenon related to shared evolutionary goals of social belonging and human connection. To live well online, the story goes, all we must do is follow our inherent desire to communicate, letting nature run its course by commenting, liking, sharing, and posting to our hearts' content. On the other hand, the normative designs of social media interfaces reveal a fundamental lack of confidence in this foundational visage. We have seen how platforms are actively involved in nudging users toward practices of busy social connection online, and how this nudging is justified through gestures toward the fallible human subject, deemed to require a little help on the way toward their own flourishing. Healthy users, then, are not actually trusted to act in their own best interests on social media. They must be guided on the path to their own well-being through liberal paternalist design interventions.

This seeming paradox can be explicated through the lens of neuroliberal governance, which has conceptually grounded the sociotechnical analysis of this book throughout. Whether working for or against users' imagined best natures, the contrasting appeals made toward evolutionary discourse and nudge architectures offer users a reason to actively engage with platforms in a manner that supposedly resonates with their own individual proclivities. These motivations, as I have argued in previous chapters, work upon and through the free actions of users, not in spite of them. As such, the inconsistent scripting of healthy users does not negate the efficacy of the governance of well-being on social media, but rather functions as part of a tangled apparatus that conducts the conduct of users for certain strategic purposes, at various points in time and space, through various means. Primarily, these contrasting motivations, and the behavioral changes they seek to encourage, effect the same ends: the continued functioning of social media as capitalist data platforms.

However, while this ties a fairly neat interpretive bow around this book's material discursive findings, it remains to be seen how users themselves situate their own social media activity and its relationship to their well-being within all of this. Do users of Facebook view their well-being on social media through the binary of active/passive use? What are the threats to their well-being they see on platforms? And do they consider their wellness habits as potential sites of self-management and self-control? To get at these questions, and to fulfill the third empirical qualitative layer of script analysis that has helped methodologically structure this book so far, I interviewed thirty-seven adult British Facebook users between September 2020 and September 2021.[1] Participants responded to physical advertisements I posted in semipublic places around the UK, in gyms, yoga studios, cafés, shops, supermarkets, and libraries for example. Participants all lived in the UK, were spread equally across gender, and varied in age, class, and ethnic backgrounds. However, all were alike in having chosen to respond, given the advertisements' stipulation that participants have a nominal interest in well-being. This initial targeted sampling method was combined with snowball sampling that utilized the existing networks of participants for subsequent interviews. The interviews took place against the backdrop of the second and third waves of UK COVID-19 lockdown measures, and all occurred remotely via video conferencing software.

The interview procedure itself involved users sharing their screen with me, logging into their Facebook, scrolling down their Feed interface, and answering questions about what we encountered. The interview began with each participant giving a "tour" of their Feed, narrating what they saw and how they would typically engage with the content they observed. Following this initial introduction, I would move on to more focused questions about what they considered healthy social media use and how they imagined the Feed to be involved in their overall well-being, if at all. This quasi–in situ technique builds on other qualitative digital methods, including Light, Burgess, and Duguay's "walkthrough method," Baym and Burgess's practice of "archival scrolling," Robards and Lincoln's technique of scrolling through the Timeline, and the "media go-along."[2]

It is perhaps obvious to say that the loosely targeted sample of this study, when combined with the specific context of the interviews, produced conversations whose significance are bounded by their own conditions. Yet the particular method I developed for this interview study sought to use this inevitable circumscription as a productive starting point, rather than a weakness. This is inspired by the thought of anthropologist Charles Briggs, who treats the interview procedure as a situated "communicative event" that creates a shared social context under the explicit pretense of creating data for subsequent analysis by the researcher.[3] The sense of circumscribed artificiality that is always and unavoidably incurred by the qualitative interview situation therefore becomes a key empirical tactic, as opposed to a barrier to understanding. Specifically, the technique of coinhabiting a usually private scrolling experience, through a focus on well-being, cultivated an explicitly fabricated tie of co-analysis between myself and the participant, prompting the users being interviewed to reflexively engage with what was a habitual, everyday activity for them. As habits are immanent to place, and often slip below conscious acknowledgment, this interview technique opened up an analytical distance between the user, the interface, and their own habits in an out-of-the-ordinary way. This step outside of the normal flow of things, somewhat counterintuitively, was precisely the thing that allowed us to examine the production, and productivity, of normative discourses and designs of habitual social media well-being *in the environment of their expression.*

Accordingly, the data created in these interviews come from situated acts of communication, growing out of the relationship between the researcher and the participant. As such, I do not claim that the findings below are objective, or neutral, or even that they offer an accurate reflection of participants' internal psyches. Moreover, the data I present below haven't been created, carved up, and analyzed in order to ascertain the one and only Truth about social media well-being for the individuals concerned (let alone being representative of a wider population). Rather, I present what follows as indications, discursive traces perhaps, of the ways that the participants were seeking to express their feelings about their well-being on social media at the time and place of the interview itself. In particular, the communicative event of each interview can be viewed as a social situation that sought to create understanding between the researcher and the participant. As such, the specific expressions users employed to extrapolate their ideas about well-being, and in particular their stated struggles with the demands of the Feed, can principally be viewed as *idioms of distress* that provide ready-at-hand shortcuts toward shared legibility.[4] I have borrowed this term from psychological anthropology, and specifically the work of Mark Nichter, who describes idioms of distress as "socially and culturally resonant means of experiencing and expressing distress in local worlds—as used specifically to foster mutual comprehension in a shared space."[5]

Developing the term in the 1980s, Nichter hoped to give a place to the influence of culture in the experience of psychiatric conditions, as a response to the expansion of psychological categories developed through Western medicalized matrices into non-Western contexts.[6] The need for such an approach relates to the insight that modalities of psychological inquiry and diagnosis are locally contingent, and are particularly entwined with Eurocentric rationalities of medicalization emergent in the Western liberal democracies of the twentieth century.[7] The implication for clinical treatment is that the relevance of psychologized interventions for experiences of mental human suffering become dependent on local circumstances, rather than being universally applicable across all contexts at all times.[8] Highlighting the situatedness of mental distress brings into focus the discursive terms through which elements of the human condition are variously constructed as problematic, very much in line with Foucauldian considerations of how the human is "made" in time through intersecting forms of normalization, subjectivation, and governance.

Nichter puts it this way: idioms of distress "are culturally constituted in the sense that they initiate particular types of interaction and are associated with culturally pervasive values, norms, generative themes, and health concerns."[9] Such *expressive modes*, as a result, "reflect not only individual suffering but also social complaints and anxieties" tied to the time and place of their articulation.[10] Thus, the in situ method of the interview technique, combined with the conceptual armature of idioms of distress, which operate on the level of situated description, will enable this chapter to take seriously the specific discursive repertoires employed by individuals to talk about problematic relations on the Feed as expressed within the environment itself. This will enable me to pay heed to the digital setting of the interview situation, exploring how its technological demands entangle with the particular backgrounds of users, the culturally resonant ways they seek to express their concerns, and how this all relates to their social milieus.

We will see how the participants spoke overwhelmingly about the Feed as a source of confusing distraction, which they did their best to limit their engagements with. We will see how they lamented the joint burdens of compulsive self-and-social comparison that the Feed was said to inculcate within them. And in response, we will see how users reflected upon the various self-nudges they had imposed on themselves to control their negative scrolling interactions. During the interviews, participants spoke about these attempts toward self-control as a losing battle, and offered sophisticated critiques as to why this was the case. Primarily, users spoke about the asymmetrical power relations involved in inhabiting an extractive platform environment that has been designed to profit from their interactions with it. Despite these well-articulated rationales for their struggles, related to the aforementioned attention economy, users spoke about the ways in which failing to control their engagements with the Feed (as they thought they should) produced painful feelings of internal guilt and public shame. Accordingly, this chapter will argue that the idioms of distress specifically related to guilt, shame, and blame used by participants to describe their Feed experience are able to identify the effects of contemporary neuroliberal responsibilization in action.

Neuroliberal *responsibilization*, to remind the reader, refers to the psychological construction and self-administration of subjects in liberal democracies, like the UK, who are encouraged to manage their own (perceived) irrational behavioral tendencies for the sake of their own well-being. Here, *well-being* boils down to the individual decision to cultivate healthy habits—well-being is constituted as simply a matter of choice. This works to divorce the individual from the material, social, and cultural conditions that support well-being, topically excluding any consideration of the social determinants of health that unevenly impact differently situated individuals inhabiting shared worlds. Against this backdrop, I argue that the idioms of social media distress channeled by participants, and the practices of self-control that accompany them, were performed in the neuroliberal style, working to trap these users within the all-too-ready-at-hand terms of responsibilization that were available at the time of the interviews. By linking the macro-level discourse of active social media well-being circulating around the UK during the interviews to its material inculcation through specific user interfaces like the Feed, and its manifestation through the expressions and activity of individual users themselves, this chapter will show how the heterogeneous elements of self-controlled social media well-being all function within apparatuses of contemporary governance and psycho-computational power.

Disrupting Habits

I began each interview by inviting participants to give me a "tour" of their Feed. This was interpreted differently by different users, but the response of Aron, a construction worker in his early twenties, illustrates a larger pattern I observed throughout the interviews. Interviewees often expressed confusion about being asked to delve into, and reflect upon, their Facebook Feed. Aron: "Yeah, sure. I can't remember the last time I actually used Facebook on a computer, which is a bit bizarre. There we go. So, there's where you post your feelings or your thoughts or what have you. There's all your events and your marketplace stuff, any shortcuts you've got. . . . [H]ere's all your stories of people you may or may not want to speak to. Yeah. That's pretty much—is that what you mean?" The open-endedness of this initial question was intended to allow participants to describe scrolling down the Feed in their own terms. I wanted to see how users would reflect on what was usually a private, habitual activity. As Aron's response demonstrates, participants were often unsure how to proceed. Both the novelty of having someone—me—watch them scroll down their Feed and doing so on a computer interface, rather than a phone, were perhaps factors in their indecision. Others, such as Erin, a translator in her mid-thirties, suggested that they had "never paid that much attention to it [their Feed], to be honest," and likewise stalled at the beginning of the interview. Through these beginnings, I began to notice how scrolling down the Feed together in this way worked to produce fabricated moments of shared analytic reflection—for both myself and the participant. Following Briggs, we can see how the artificial interview situation ruptured users' normal scrolling practice—*creating* data on the Feed, rather than simply gathering it.

Following this initial tour of the Feed, I then invited participants to scroll down the interface more freely, narrating what they saw along the way. Some, like Dan, a glass worker in his early thirties, were cautious, asking, "What do you want us to go through, and what do you want to know?" Others, like Sharon, a retired social worker in her mid-sixties, were more forthcoming in their descriptions:

So, what I tend to do is look at the things from my friends, and then most of the things I'll just scroll by because there's so much crap on Facebook now. So, I used to use it quite a lot, but I've been using it increasingly less as time goes by. I know my daughter's using Instagram more than Facebook. A lot of the youngsters are not using it as much anymore, but I just don't want to be fucking around with another app. So, I'll look at things from my friends, and then if I come across—sometimes I'll see adverts. I see something about Greenpeace now, which I find quite interesting, so I might open that up and see what they're talking about, which is fine. So, I presume that there are algorithms that have kind of identified that I'm interested in environmental issues. That's fine. I've got friends who post constantly, and it's a lot of waffle, so I'll just zoom past them and ignore it, or I might press the "like" just to be polite.

As I began coding and analyzing participants' opening salvos, I found that although the content of each user's Feed was qualitatively unique, and levels of description varied, the way scrolling through this content was described as a distraction was remarkably similar. Primarily, scrolling was spoken about as an effort of resisting the Feed's attentive demands. Participants described the Feed as a space of diversion, sometimes trivial, sometimes traumatic, but always captivating. Users described this odd stranglehold as being linked to experiencing the Feed as a fluid concoction of content—a random blend of ideas, news articles, friends, family, adverts, memories, images, videos, and the rest. For example, Jaxon, a freelance video editor in his late twenties, described the Feed as "a strange mix" during his tour:

I feel like it's just all a lot of information in your face in one go. . . . There's just a lot of things. There's a lot of information. You don't really know. Oh. Someone else with a baby. You don't really know—

you don't really know where to look and what's really—and I think actually for me the main stressor point that I have with social media is I feel, like, because you're scrolling like this really quickly, there's a lot of information, you just move on really—you just learn to move on really quickly and I think it's just that. That definitely impacts my concentration levels when it comes to other things.

Jaxon's comments echo the majority of those interviewed, who often indicated that they felt disorientated and troubled when interacting with the Feed at length.

Leon, a charity worker in his mid-thirties, found the Feed "quite horrible to look at," saying that he was "conscious that I'm just being bombarded with content" while scrolling through it. Leon went on to say that if he spent extended periods of time on the Feed, he experienced a "weird feeling": "It's kind of like—it's like a steady loss of attention span, I think. For me, it's this weird almost like panicky hyperactivity where I could feel myself not being able to concentrate on one thing for more than like two minutes." In a similar vein, Tobi, early thirties, unemployed and on state benefits, described the Feed as "unpredictable," observing that "you will get the most banal, trivial, jokey kinds of comments from people, and the next thing down will be like someone talking about the most serious kind of brutal stories, of current affairs, and things that are really kind of depressing and serious. And it's like getting those two things, like one after the other, and it's just mixed up to that extent. I think that's kind of a strange thing about it." This, for Tobi, can "elicit an emotional response that you're not looking for," which he claimed he did not "really enjoy." As Tobi's and Leon's comments illustrate, participants described the Feed as a flowing stream of content that discombobulated, distracted, and diverted their attention, in manners and directions that were not always deemed pleasant.

Idioms of Social Media Distress

As outlined above, it is useful to think of these negative descriptions of the Feed as idioms of distress. For Nichter, who first coined the term, idioms of distress are situated expressions "based far more on presentation and negotiation than on static representations," reflecting multiple temporal scales at once that entwine past and "contemporary life" within the contextual environments of their articulation.[11] In this case, participants were describing the Feed as a drain of their attention, and often linked this to broader concerns about the dangers of the so-called attention economy. That many of the participants were doing so is perhaps not surprising. At the time of the interviews, and as further discussed in the introduction of this book, the well-being dangers of "toxic" social media platforms were under intense public scrutiny, being frequently discussed in newspapers and magazines, in documentaries, and on public service broadcasters like the BBC. The ways in which platforms were said to profit from outrage, hateful content, polarization, and the capturing and denigration of attention in general were a major part of the so-called "tech-lash" that was whipping around the broader mediatized horizon of the UK at the time.[12]

During his interview, for instance, Dan provided a rationale behind his struggle for attention on the Feed: "That's what it's for, isn't it? It grabs your attention, and it pulls you in it. That's why there are these suggested posts, to keep you online, to keep you going through it, to keep you clicking through stuff." Like Dan, other participants said they were well aware of the pernicious designs of social media like Facebook, and how this could impact their attention in particular. Some of the participants explicitly referenced the documentary *The Social Dilemma* to discuss how the design of the Feed inculcated repetitious behaviors that distracted them from other tasks. Laura, a journalist in her late thirties, likened it to video gambling machines: "I do know that it's designed to be like slot machines. You're just trying to pull from more and more. The never-ending timeline is, like, *the thing*, you know, you can just spend all day on it. And you know there's more content there, you just have to scroll—the tease of all that." Laura's use of the word *tease* suggests enticement from the Feed, persuasion, desire. Saying that you "*have* to scroll" hints at its strong allure.

Geoff, a software engineer working for a nonprofit organization, in his mid-thirties, saw all of this as a battle, as a fight for his agency. Interestingly, Geoff presents a similar view of fallible human psychology found in nudge to describe how his behavior was being manipulated on the Feed, as explored in chapter 2: "I understand, as a consumer of Facebook's product, I am fighting hundreds of amazing user experience and design engineers who are very good at capitalizing on the habitual nature of human psychology [to keep me scrolling]." As we can see, these users all adopted similar terms to express how the Feed negatively targeted their behavior and attention. This could reflect the way that attention, in the words of Morton Axel Pedersen and colleagues, "has become a prominent source of moral anxiety and cultural imagination in the twenty-first century—an issue around which ethical, political, and economic discourses and practices congeal."[13] Indeed, expressions of how best to "spend" one's attention are inextricably linked to the hegemonic discourses and designs of social media well-being we have encountered in this book so far.[14] Moreover, the demand to control personal attention and the stated need for focus when engaging with social media are very much reflective of the broader discourses and designs of neuroliberal governance discussed in previous chapters. In particular, the type of behavioral self-management that engagement with the Feed seemingly required from these participants (1) subjectified them as users that were fallible to distraction and (2) inculcated behaviors within them that produced them as such. Here, we can see how adopting this stance toward the Feed produces users of a certain style, trapped within the discursive terms of the attention economy and limited to neuroliberal tactics of atomized behavioral transformation in response.

Accordingly, the idioms of distress employed by users to describe the impact of the Feed on their attention indicate that participants were perhaps grasping at what Raymond Williams might have termed *structures of feeling*—shifts in "presence" and "pressures" felt and described by individuals within changing mediatized sociopolitical environments, at specific historical junctures.[15] However, rather than treat these references to attention as reflective of measurable, categorizable states of being, I believe it is yet more fruitful to examine how participants employ such terms in response to the Feed environment itself, for what purposes, and pertaining to what effects. In other words, I examine what these specific idioms of social media distress allowed users to say, and what they did not. As we will see throughout this chapter, it is in these particular discrepancies of expression, and the styles of conduct they delimit, that the politics of social media well-being can be found.

Normative Comparison

After these opening narrations, I asked participants to expand upon the feelings they had expressed in relation to the attentive pull of the Feed. Overall, participants described how they struggled to manage the emotional impact that scrolling down the Feed had on them. The rapid flow of content led to contrasting feelings of emptiness and despair, of titillation and joy, all felt in quick succession. While the loss of attention was something that all participants were worried about, another major concern for participants was how the Feed led to practices of social comparison. In one sense, the Feed was seen to divert attention in random directions. In another sense, however, it also directed users' attention toward unasked-for, yet personally relevant, anxiety-inducing topics. That is, in bringing participants closer to the lives of other users in their personal milieus—whatever that specifically meant in terms of age, ethnicity, profession, class, and so on for each user—scrolling down the Feed inculcated practices of comparison, which in turn brought them closer to the operative norms of their individual social worlds. This is something Alice Marwick has explored as a form of social surveillance, whereby the visibility of interaction on the Feed produces networks of mutually reciprocated user discipline.[16] The well-being impacts of this social comparison are also a prevalent concern of the psychological literature, as identified in the introduction. During the interviews, it was possible to see how similar discursive formations of normalization were always lurking behind the idioms of social media distress expressed by the participants. This section will specifically show how users expressed feelings of personal guilt and social shame whenever they viewed themselves as failing to live up to the perceived requirements of their imagined social existence.

Even though all participants believed that the lives on show on the Feed constituted a "highlight" reel, and perhaps did not represent actual lived mundanity, participants spoke about how being confronted with such presentations nevertheless made them reflect negatively on their own life circumstances as a result.[17] For Eve, a yoga teacher in her mid-thirties, this came down to the layout of the Feed interface, which she felt was "designed to have you compare yourself to others." Eve continued: "So, what I notice is that when I go on social media, if I'm in a good mood, I'm having a nice day, I can scroll maybe three or four times, and somehow, I just don't feel good anymore. I don't feel good about myself. I don't feel good about my life. And I find that strange because ten minutes before I scrolled, I felt fine." Likewise, for Erin, the damaging impact of the Feed's comparative pull meant that if she spent too long on the Feed she began to feel "overwhelmed" and that she needed to "step back" from it at regular intervals. In the field of science and technology studies, Joe Deville, Michael Guggenheim, and Zuzana Hrdličková describe *comparison* as "processes of calibration," a "holding steady" of the world "just long enough for questions of difference and similarity to come into view."[18] The Feed invited those I interviewed to hold steady their own life in relation to the idealized lives of others. This calibrating process entangled them with the operative norms of their own world, bringing them closer to their imagined expectations and felt pressures, three examples of which I will turn to now.

Tobi said that the type of content he saw scrolling down his Feed made him reflect upon his unemployed status in a negatively comparative way, perhaps as a response to British classist hegemony surrounding the individualized shame of being out of work.[19] Tobi said he

was aware that when I'm sitting at home and its lockdown, and it's raining, and I'm unemployed, I shouldn't be looking through people's holiday photo albums . . . because ultimately, you end up comparing yourself to what you're looking at, [even though] what you're looking at is not an accurate representation of somebody else's life. So, you're comparing your state of happiness and enjoyment while you're staring at your Facebook Feed. And let's face it, you're never going to be staring at your Facebook Feed while you're having the time of your life. So, you kind of compare yourself to people, images of people, where they're having the time of their lives. And that's a recipe for feeling a little bit down about your state, the state of your life, in a way.

Farah, an account manager in her late thirties who had a young daughter, spoke about comparing herself to other mothers' presentations of family life on the Feed. While we were scrolling, Farah encountered a subgroup of her local mothering group: "Oh, that's another group that I'm in . . . where it's people suggesting days out with young families. Looking at that can be like, 'Oh gosh have I been out enough? Have I taken her [Farah's daughter] to this place or that place?' And then I feel guilty if I haven't done that. Those kinds of feelings stir up." For Farah, then, the Feed invited her to consider her identity as a mother, and whether she was stacking up against other families, possibly revelatory of operative ideals of gendered and nuclear assumptions of motherhood.[20]

Joy, a yoga teacher in her mid-forties, spoke at length about her struggles with Facebook, and how it worsened her ongoing battles with self-esteem. Joy described how she had, in the past, compared herself with other members of the running and yoga groups she was part of on Facebook. This was often detrimental to her mood: "I'd be like, 'Oh, my god. My running's not fast enough. Everybody's faster than me. Oh, my god. My yoga poses aren't as good as everybody else's. Oh, my god. My body doesn't look like everybody else's.' And it was getting to the point where it was causing me more grief than enjoyment, being on there." The Feed's comparative tendencies manifested for Joy in the way she measured herself against other fitness enthusiasts, perhaps revealing the competitive dimensions of quantified self movements, or dominant Western imaginations of the (white) ideal yoga body type.[21]

These examples are obviously short and undeveloped. You could write an entire book on their respective dimensions and the politics to be found therein if you wanted to. However, I want to focus instead on how the Feed, in the words of Taina Bucher, gave Tobi, Farah, and Joy each a "reason to react."[22] Am I a valuable member of society? Am I a good mother? Am I physically fit enough? The motivation behind, content of, and answers to these types of questions are obviously relative and unique to the life circumstance and personality of each participant. Yet it is the shared dynamic and conjoined process of asking them at all—and how they relate to, reinforce, or challenge the specifics of comparison—that is most important here. The norms presented on the Feed elicited a reaction from users. Therefore, whether accepted or not, we can see how comparative practices on the Feed nevertheless made these norms present, salient, and felt. Participants did not describe this form of normative comparison on the Feed as an active choice, or even as something they would want to do at all. Rather, the Feed, as outlined above, was imagined as inculcating these practices of comparison whether participants liked it or not.

Participants also frequently spoke about comparing themselves against past versions of their own selves on the Feed, in a way that likewise opened opportunities for sometimes uncanny reflections and self-doubt. During her interview, for example, Emma, a physical therapist in her early forties, spoke about the conflicting feelings she had when she saw posts from friends who lived in a city she no longer lived in. She wondered out loud why she hadn't deleted these contacts, even though she hadn't spoken to them in years. After some deliberation, Emma went on to suggest that it felt too "final to just cut people out." Emma described her life then, and her mixed feelings about being reminded of it on the Feed:

> I was doing a PhD, and I was doing fieldwork in the tropics and life was quite exciting in a lot of ways. There was all this future ahead of me and lots of promise for the future. And things did work out in the direction I'd hoped, to an extent. But they also swung back in a different direction afterwards as well. And things never pan out exactly as you expect, I suppose. So, when I think back to then it's very mixed. There's part of me that wants to hang on to how I was feeling then, what I was doing then, the stuff that was going on in my life, and the people, and stay in touch. But there's another part of me that, with the benefit of hindsight, can look at it and it can feel a little painful.

Because I didn't know what was coming at that time. Not that something terrible happened, but I ended up leaving academia. I ended up going in a very different direction and there was just a general upheaval. So perhaps there's a part of me that wonders if it would be easier to not be reminded all the time of these past incarnations of myself.

Likewise, Tobi spoke of the way scrolling down the Feed for a bit of "benign entertainment" can often quickly twist into something more troubling. Like Emma, Tobi felt "involuntarily exposed to old memories of old times without really wanting to visit those memories." Tobi said this "will lead me to have melancholy thoughts because it will provoke me to think about the past. Sometimes I've even kind of realized I'm having these thoughts and I'll just quickly close Facebook and say, 'Why the hell am I looking at this?'" Whereas Lee Humphreys demonstrates how the personal cultivation of memories on social media could form part of active self-narrativizations, Emma's and Tobi's comments do not suggest that these frequent trips down memory lane on Facebook were actually chosen or, indeed, wanted.[23]

Addiction and Technological Guilt

When I interviewed Samuel, a charity worker in his mid-forties, COVID lockdown measures in England were in full effect. Perhaps because of this, Samuel was especially reflective, and sometimes somber, during his interview. Recalling the critiques of the attention economy outlined previously in this book, he argued that the Feed is "designed to stimulate you." In Samuel's case, the Feed brought him closer to the personal and national devastation of COVID. He reported this as being detrimental to his mood, yet strangely intoxicating:

Say in the pandemic . . . every day I look at the numbers and the stats, and then I look at the news. And I had to restrict looking at that. Because it's on your phone or whatever. You can just pick it up at any time, and just see what's going on right now. And you can't do anything about it, and it's actually really overwhelming. If you're just constantly looking at it, it's draining. It's so negative, but it becomes hard to stop. It's hard to pull yourself away from that. I think it does become quite addictive.

Here, Samuel uses an idiom of distress related to addiction to describe his habitual relationship to the Feed. Addiction was a prominent metaphor used in this way by almost all the participants, including Farah, who put it more strongly (as quoted in this chapter's first epigraph): "Fundamentally, I dislike Facebook. I would probably go so far as saying I actually hate it. But that doesn't stop me going on it every single day, probably three to four times a day." Farah, like many others interviewed, described the looming presence of the Feed as something they were beholden to, stating it was "addictive," and "it's got power over me." As I have argued throughout the book, discourses of digital addiction tend to turn the psychic distress experienced via technology inward, blaming the individual for failure to control their use, mood, and interactions in digital spheres, negating any consideration of the wider material, political, environmental, and social circumstances that those moods and behaviors are relating to and within which they are expressed. Nevertheless, and echoing similar findings by Katrin Tiidenberg and colleagues, discourses of addiction were widely circulating in mediatized discussions of social media well-being at the time of the interviews, implicitly mobilizing subject/object divisions between users and machines, and of the controller and the controlled.[24] Perhaps in response to this, participants frequently invoked descriptions of addiction, along with corresponding similes of other vices, to talk about their struggles of overuse during the interviews.

Most significant here is how these descriptions were often accompanied by idioms of distress relating to guilt, confessed by those participants who imagined themselves unable to practice necessary restraint on the Feed. Jaxon, for example, stated, "It's like a drug that you know you shouldn't be doing, but you're doing it anyway." Employing a similarly loaded comparison, Mia, a yoga teacher in her mid-thirties, described social media as her "vice": "I will be honest, social media is my vice. Other people have alcohol and stuff like that. Social media is mine. So, I do feel like people can have a healthy relationship with it, but I think it does take a lot of self-discipline for that to happen." Here, Mia reiterates a discourse of self-discipline and self-regulation that other participants frequently employed during the interviews. For other participants, there was a sense that uncontrolled use of the Feed was a wrongdoing, and this frequently coalesced around certain scrolling habits. For instance, Chelsea, in her early thirties and working in finance, said, "I'm definitely guilty of using my phone as an alarm clock. Which means that I'm taking it [the Feed] in and checking it first thing in the morning, when I wake up. That's something that I have thought I'd like to cut down on." Some participants attached judgments of laziness to others' and their own perceived failure to control their social media habits.

This contrasting of "lazy" and "active" habits, which map onto norms of "bad" and "good" respectively, find one parallel in the mediatized treatment of fatness in Western domains, as examined by Deborah Lupton.[25] Lupton argues that such stigmatization functions within broader processes of neoliberal health (non)intervention, hailing indolent subjects imagined to be incapable of self-care, and who ought to be governed as such. Julie Guthman has examined this elsewhere in terms of *healthism*, which "makes personal health attainment the highest goal, sees poor health outcomes as a result of behaviors, and conflates personal practices of self-care with empowerment and good citizenship."[26] Guthman similarly relates this to "neoliberal norms of governance" insofar as it "concedes the roll-back of public-sector responsibility for supporting and protecting the health of all and instead places responsibility on individuals for their own health outcomes."[27]

For example, Ava, a personal trainer in her mid-thirties, provided a telling comparison of this process in operation (as quoted in this chapter's second epigraph). Saying that Facebook is "really addictive" and designed to be so, she blamed the "quite lazy" addicts themselves, "because it's kind of like obese people saying that it's McDonald's' fault for them eating too many McDonald's." Ava concluded that only "a tiny portion of the fault is with Facebook." In a less outwardly judgmental vein, Emma switched her critique inward, calling herself "lazy" for not curating her friends on Facebook: "I know a lot of people are much more on it in terms of cropping their friends, and kind of keeping it down to a small group. I'm incredibly lazy in that regard." More softly, Dina, a retiree in her mid-sixties, spoke about her husband teasing her for constantly checking social media on her phone when they were together. She claimed, or admitted, "I probably do use it [Facebook] more often than I should." Here, users were describing their attempts to control their scrolling habits as something they "should" be doing, calling it a "vice" and feeling "guilty" and "lazy" for failing to do so.

The painful moral failings associated with unconscious use were deemed by users to be all their own fault. That is, if they were struggling online, users explained this as being a result of their not personally doing enough to resist the damaging pull of the Feed. If struggling, they had failed themselves. We will return to the effects of this guilt, shame, and blame in the final sections of this chapter and clarify their overlapping conceptual parameters. However, for now we will focus on the responsibility users felt toward controlling their interactions with the Feed, in order to avoid its potentially negative well-being impacts, and what steps they had taken to protect themselves from such outcomes. Muhammad, a special educational needs assistant in his early twenties, emphasized the personal responsibility of users throughout his interview. Muhammad suggested that engaging with the Feed requires "self-regulation." He spoke about his efforts toward this end, arguing that "you've got to put sanctions in place . . . so you're not getting too overwhelmed" by the platform. Muhammad said that it was not only important for him but also for others to "know when you may be on it [the Feed] too much." Channeling the discourses of responsibilization discussed in previous chapters, and echoing the neuroliberal nudges frequently found in the popular self-help literature, it was important for Muhammad to make "little changes, like switching off the notifications on your phone" to gain back some control over social media. These little hacks were something that many other participants readily spoke about during the interviews. The following section will detail what these practices looked like in more depth.

Self-Nudges

The interviewees described numerous tactics whereby they sought to control their engagements with the Feed, as well as their access to social media in general. Chief among these were practices of notification management, adopting habits of mindful use, creating barriers to social media access, and cultivating a positive Feed environment. This section will present each of these practices in turn and argue that they ought to be understood as self-nudges that produce users within neuroliberal regimes of governance. Here, users were arranging their interactions with the Feed as if they were conscious *choice architects* of their own activity, replicating discourses of nudge that view the manipulation of the environment as a key lever of healthy behavioral change in the present day.

Notification Controls

Notifications were often described by participants as gateways to the Feed, which could then lead to more prolonged, detrimental, periods of scrolling. Chelsea, for example, highlighted the red color of the notification bell as part of its allure: "It's sort of a warning kind of a color. It's the color of danger." Similarly, Leon: "I don't know anything about evolutionary biology or anything like that, but red is like an alert. Right? It grabs your attention." Following the widely disseminated critiques targeted at the "addictive" design of Facebook, most notably expressed by the Center for Humane Technology, for example, these participants appeared to be interpreting the attraction of notifications through ready-at-hand associations made between the color red and what this color apparently signals to the evolutionarily conceived human brain. As such, many of the participants saw turning off notifications for the Feed as a key strategy in maintaining a distance from it. Aron, for example, said he turned off his notifications because he didn't want to be "lulled in" to scrolling the Feed by responding to them.

Mindful Use

Work by Nancy Baym and colleagues indicates that many Facebook users in the United States adopt vocabularies of mindful scrolling to talk about how they try and manage their interactions with the platform, perhaps drawing from New Age wellness discourses.[28] Similarly, the UK users I interviewed spoke of mindful engagement with their Feeds as a technique to ameliorate the potential overwhelm of undirected scrolling practice. For example, Nadia, who openly discussed the relationship between her social media use and her mental health, spoke of trying to use the Feed with a "purpose," while Joy spoke about "intentional" use of the interface. For Joy, this meant trying to be conscious of how they communicated with others on the Feed. Rather than immediately react to the posts that anger her, Joy said she would instead "take a pause, take a breath, and think, 'Okay. Do I need to respond to that?' And if I do, [I think,] 'How is that just either going to support whatever's going off or incite more issues?'" Many of the people interviewed, especially those with meditation or yoga practices, reported this type of self-reflective engagement as a method to improve their relationship with the Feed. The relationship between such discourses of mindfulness and neoliberal individualization has been examined before.[29] It is pertinent that these views expressed by users very much chime with Meta's call for conscious engagement as one key to digital wellness, which we have explored in this book so far.

For other participants, mindful use of the Feed constituted being aware of when they were scrolling, and in what company. Harry, a civil servant in his early forties, spoke about him "doing that habitual thing of picking my phone up and checking it every ten minutes,"

> And I hate [it]—I genuinely have to make conscious decisions to stop doing that. . . . It was like, "I'm not immersed in this experience, I am with somebody else but I'm glued to the News Feed," and I just—it really just resonated with me that it was a really bad way to live my life, and I wasn't giving 100 percent of myself to the people that I was with. I was glued to the stupid phone.

Other users likewise spoke about the importance of avoiding "phubbing," understood as ignoring conversational partners in social situations in favor of scrolling through one's phone, due to its damaging effects on their relationships.[30] Rob, a warehouse worker in his thirties, for example, said he and his partner had made a "conscious decision" to not use social media in each other's company because it felt like "time not very well spent." Mindful use, for these participants, therefore constituted both styles of social media interaction and the situations they would allow that activity to take place within.

Barriers of Access

To enable this type of conscious engagement with the Feed, participants discussed a range of barriers they had put in place to limit their access to Facebook. Along with removing Feed notifications, Laura, for example, reported that she had moved her social media applications on a phone to a folder titled "Once a Day." This slight diversion, for Laura, meant that her use of Facebook became a choice, rather than an unconscious obligation: "I'm choosing to interact with it. I'm going to spend this time interacting with it, rather than letting it pop up and suck me into it throughout the day." Emma had similarly moved her Facebook application to a folder labeled "Attention Parasites." When asked why she had named it in this way, Emma replied, "To remind me how I sometimes feel about it. And so, when I decide I want to look at it, I have to consciously go through a few pages, just a few more swipes and then two clicks to get into it and be confronted with that heading." Using the language of nudge explored in previous chapters, we can see how some users were providing themselves with a space for reflection before they decided to access their social media accounts. Here, interrupting the flow of fast, unconscious, habitual scrolling activity was presented by Laura and Emma as efforts to foster more considered thinking that could lead to making "better" choices with the Feed. As such, following the framework of nudge, we could view this as an attempt by these users to support their imagined-to-be long-term rational thinking, so-called System 2 cognition, over the more impulsive varieties of System 1 thinking. Some participants, however, reported that they had deleted the application from their phone completely, which George found a "big help" in his stated attempts to limit his scrolling habits. With these types of interventions, it seems, users were intervening in their own digital environment on their own behalf, responding to their own imagined-to-be unthinking nature and their inability to resist the pull of the Feed. In this way, these users presented themselves as if they were choice architects of their own behaviors on Facebook, performing the role of the neuroliberal subject of nudge in their understanding of, and attempts to manage, their well-being on the Feed.

Nadia spoke candidly about the correlation she saw between her increased social media use and her worsening mental health. Nadia suggested she had tried several of the techniques outlined above to stem her use of Facebook, and also Instagram, including deleting both applications off her phone. When I asked why she had done so, Nadia replied that "it was making me miserable":

> I would go to both Facebook and Instagram looking for connection, and after I was getting really depressed. And I sort of did a bit of a pulse check in a way. . . . I would be using these and find myself getting more and more miserable and detached, and I would feel more lonely. So I'd go on thinking I'm going to connect to people, and come away feeling a lot lonelier, so I recognized this and decided to delete them from my phone.

Nadia's comments echo those made by others above, revealing how participants were often using idioms of distress related to loneliness and depression to describe the effects of scrolling down the Feed, and how cutting it out of their lives completely was seen as one of the only ways to mitigate its negative effects.

Curating the Environment

Some users saw cultivating a positive Feed environment as a key technique to safeguard against reported feelings of loneliness, depression, and overwhelm, again chiming with Meta's call for users to inhabit an "inspiring" Feed. Harry did so because he believed that "you are a product of your environment" and that it was users' responsibility to "curate" their Feed:

> You are completely accountable and responsible for what you curate. And I'm not sure if a lot of people are aware that they have that responsibility themselves or have the strength of mind to differentiate between what's positive and what's negative, and what's potentially making them feel bad. And having that strength of character to remove yourself sometimes from the things that don't make you feel good. . . . [S]ometimes that takes a bit of personal resilience to do that, to just cut that kind of—almost cut that disease out of your life and go, "No. It's affecting my mindset and where I am as a human being. That's not good for my well-being."

Echoing Ava's comments about user addiction and obesity, Harry thus spoke of personal strength, resilience, and decision as the primary safeguards against the potential harms of the Feed. Accordingly, Harry stated that he was very selective about whom and what he interacted with on Facebook, often utilizing the snooze, unfollow, hide, or report function to tailor his Feed to his preferences. Within Harry's account, we can also witness a strong example of how the responsibilization of social media well-being produces a moral economy of blame to circulate throughout the issue. That is, if you are struggling with your well-being on social media, the implication is that you simply haven't taken the necessary measures to look after yourself and manage your activity online. Users are at fault if they are not doing this; users are to blame if they are struggling with their use of platforms.

Hanna, an accountant in her mid-twenties, was perhaps the least concerned about her Facebook use out of all the participants. Hanna actively kept her Facebook friend list to one hundred people or fewer. She did this through deleting friends she no longer spoke to "in real life." Hanna: "I think it's down to about once a year now I do a cull, just to kind of keep numbers down." During his interview, Dan likewise described having recently had "a big dump of friends" on Facebook. When asked why he did that, Dan gave a different reason: "It's just I'm not interested in what people that I don't know are posting, do you know what I mean? That's not relevant in my life, so why do I need to see it? Yeah, just posting daft videos of stuff that either gets your gripe or horrible things or stuff to do with cancer all the time, like depressing stuff. You don't want that in your life, so you get rid of it." In this way, the friend cull was interpreted as being able to prune the Feed of its attentive allure, or remove negative, "depressing" content.

Choice Architects of the Self

The type of psychological self-hacking and environmental manipulation found in these four categories of nudge expands neuroliberal governance onto new empirical terrains. Whereas, in classic liberal paternalism, external choice architects are the ones who nudge the collective to make healthier decisions through subtle interventions, these interview data reveal how individual users were nudging themselves to support "better" personal engagements with their Feeds. Crucially, these users all implied that they were doing so to improve and work upon their own imagined psychological fallibility. Users all spoke about how, if they could control their engagements with the Feed, they wouldn't need to put these measures in place to help them. As such, the entrepreneur of the self of classic neoliberalism is now joined on the scene by a neuroliberal choice architect of the self, consciously self-hacking themselves, and their own perceived ineptitude, toward better decisions and healthier choices in the digital realm.[31] In doing so, these users were describing their well-being on social media as a result of their own choices alone. This is not an insignificant or neutral insight. Instead, as I have demonstrated at length in previous sections, the focus on personal choice isolates people from their social context, ratifying meritocratic myths as correct heuristics for the interpretation of social media well-being. By inhabiting the neuroliberal subject position of nudge, these participants, whether consciously or not, were operationalizing discourses of responsibilization that were prevalent in the UK at the time of the interviews, and that have been dominant in the public imaginary in the neoliberalized Global North for at least the past forty years.

This is not to ascribe fault to these users for doing so, or even to suggest that they were simply blind to the political implications of this stance. As we will see below, some users were keen to link these feelings of self-blame to wider apparatuses of power in their interviews. Rather, it is interesting that despite the critical knowledge that blaming themselves and other users for negative Feed experiences was not really helpful, or accurate, the vocabulary users most readily grasped for to describe their experiences nevertheless came from the language of nudge. This could indicate that the connection between behavioral psychology and social media well-being, which this book has shown to be mutually supporting, is now so pervasive that expressing the issue in any other terms has become difficult. Expressing oneself beyond the purview of nudge, that is, was perhaps implicitly seen as a barrier to shared understanding within the communicative event of the interview situation itself. Overall, the idioms of social media distress employed by users were saturated with neoliberal tropes and neuroliberal discourse, indicating that such repertoires offered a way for their concerns to be heard, to be understood, at the time of the interview, at the particular place of its staging.

In this way, following Raymond Williams once more, perhaps we can describe the focus on digital self-control displayed by these participants as a currently hegemonic structure of feeling, insofar as it relates to

> a whole body of practices and expectations, over the whole of living; our senses and assignments of energy, our shaping perceptions of ourselves and our world. It is a lived system of meanings and values— constitutive and constituting—which as they are experienced as practices appear as reciprocally confirming. It thus constitutes a sense of reality for most people in the society, a sense of absolute because experienced reality beyond which it is very difficult for most members of the society to move, in most areas of their lives.[32]

Considering the neuroliberal dimensions of nudge, and its distinctly political implications, you may wonder if we should so easily accept its language to describe social media well-being in this way. Given that structures of feeling are in no way fixed, and remain open to new interpretations, new links to the past, and new links to what it means to be a human existing as part of a community of others, it may be time to collectively imagine alternative standpoints for us to adopt, perhaps ones that do not so readily target and blame individual users for their perceived behavioral shortcomings online. This book's conclusion will provide a route to this end, while the next section will further outline the many obstacles in the way.

Connected Obligation

If the Feed caused these users so much trouble, you may be beginning to ask, why didn't they just quit? When situated within the expanding literature on digital disconnection explored in earlier sections of this book, this question becomes a bit more tricky. As Zeena Feldman has specifically highlighted, whether or not users choose to connect with social media is not really a case of either/or.[33] Rather, for some users, ambivalent entanglement with social media demonstrates a *beyond-choice ontology*, "where digital participation is regarded as a necessity rather than a choice."[34] Among those I interviewed, given the perceived beyond-choice status of the Feed, which had become crucial to their sociality, family relationships, and job prospects, all they could do was limit the Feed's damaging effects as best they could. As outlined above, users described an armory of self-management techniques they had adopted to handle the Feed's felt necessity. In the words of Pearl, a massage therapist in her mid-fifties, and echoing the tool-view of technology presented in the introduction, the self-nudges explored above were understood as a way for users "to feel in control" of the Feed, "rather than it controlling" them.

This struggle for control was not described as an easy task. Every user interviewed described their drive for self-discipline on the Feed as a losing battle, a rigged game. Mia, for example, claimed that "you should be able to have the discipline" on the Feed, "but, also, it's not set up for discipline, is it? Social media is not set up for bounded use. It's there to be used as much as possible. That's why they keep making it as user-friendly as possible." Here, Mia touches upon a core tension expressed by the participants during the interviews: How to resist the harmful pull of the Feed against the technological arsenal of its capitalist creators? Geoff phrased this tension in a rich response, again relating his inability to control his use of the Feed in terms of his own psychological fallibility:

> I unfollowed literally everybody on my friends list. There's no one who got special treatment. Everyone was unfollowed. So, when the inevitable reflex to load Facebook up happened, I didn't have anything interesting to look at, and I would do something else. It's ridiculous. You're having to set up these little psychological escapes for yourself because you know full well you're going to get pulled back

in. It's like fighting your own instincts that are being played by a bunch of UX engineers in California. It's so annoying. But that's the only way I've found—because just deleting it completely, you can't do that because too many people use Facebook to get in touch with you.

As these comments further reveal, users were well aware of the digital "traps" of social media as examined by Nick Seaver, and understood their asymmetric position within the imagined attention economy within which they were laid.[35]

In this way, users reported that quitting their Feed was not a realistic option, due to both its attentive pull and its being essential to their lives in some way. Lucas, for example, a risk assessment manager in his mid-thirties, spoke about how the Feed was necessary for him to keep in contact with his tabletop-gaming social groups in the city where he lived. Lucas described how gaming tournaments were organized only on Facebook, "so if you don't get on it and get yourself a slot," Lucas said, "you're going to miss out." This, coupled with Lucas's desire to keep in contact with friends who lived internationally, led him to describe the Feed as "an essential utility for interacting with people." Lucas maintained this belief despite his description of Facebook as a "monster" that he would gladly delete if he only thought it was possible. Likewise, Laura, a US citizen living in the UK, suggested that Facebook was one of the only methods she had to keep in touch with her family overseas: "The various times I've thought about deleting my Facebook, it would for me personally would feel like I would actually just be cutting off the only connection I have to friends and family."

Relatedly, Bobby, an academic and father in his mid-sixties, claimed that his phone was a proxy for the various social connections that it facilitated, and that losing it often felt like a loss of those relationships. For Bobby, this sometimes led to panic:

If I don't know where my phone is, it's like suddenly you start patting your pockets and start going "Oh shit, where is it?" Because it's a communication thing, and so with my son, and the kids, and the family, this is how we communicate, and how we keep in touch. So, if I lose that, then I kind of lose the family, or lose the friends, or lose whatever. So, it's that. It is an interesting concept that this thing in my pocket represents my connection, my social connections to those others. I realize that I am wedded to it, and I try to pretend that I'm not, but I know I am.

Bobby introduces a notion of being "wedded" to his device to supplement the idioms of distress relating to addiction employed by other participants. Both terms suggest a sense of duty, of obligation. Such sentiments appeared as recurring themes throughout the interviews. Yet duty toward the Feed was felt in different ways for participants, especially for those who, unlike Bobby, were not in stable employment at the time of their interview. For example, during his interview, Jaxon, a freelance video editor, spoke about regularly disabling his Facebook account due to its being a drain on his attention. However, he never went as far as to delete it completely, as he didn't want to "lose a line of communication" with people in his industry who used Facebook, or lose access to "job pages" relevant for his profession. Likewise, Elsie, a part-time waitress in her late twenties who was looking for permanent work in the cultural sector at the time of her interview, spoke about using the Feed to keep her up-to-date with relevant events and workshops that could benefit her career. Elsie used the Feed to find useful "job information" and felt that deleting it would cut her off from these links to more secure employment. Interacting with the Feed, therefore, was a literal networking activity for these users, necessary for their respective employment hopes.

For those with small businesses, furthermore, the Feed was viewed as a necessary space for promotion and advertisement. Eve, for example, who part-owned the yoga studio where she also taught, illustrates this point: "Social media is linked to my survival. If I don't participate, I won't make money. I can't make a living. That's really bad. That's really bad, because we don't have any other ways of advertising. . . . There's a big gap there that I don't know how to bridge, unless I stay very, very local in my life and start knocking on people's doors." Nadia, a self-employed yoga teacher, summarized it like this: "part and parcel of being self-employed is you have to go where the people are, and the people are on Facebook, unfortunately." As Ulrich Dolata explains, these sentiments reveal how platforms such as Facebook now "constitute, organize, and regulate competitive conditions and market contexts," imbricating the business practices of individuals and groups with the technological demands and profit motives of the environment itself.[36] Therefore, when we think about the imagined obligation of the Feed, it is important to note how this is felt differently by different users depending on their personal circumstances.

Well-Being as Balance

Overall, participants spoke about their well-being on Facebook, and in technological spheres more broadly, as part of a holistic set of shifting relations between the self, technology, others, the environment, and the cultural, social, and political world around them. The participants suggested that balancing these various relations in harmony was the key to their well-being in a general sense, with well-being in the digital realm understood as part of this broader spectrum, rather than as a discrete concept. For some of the participants, this holistic notion of well-being existed in tension with the vision of social media well-being as an outcome of individual choice, as implied within the discourses of self-nudge introduced above. The closing sections of this chapter will explore this tension in more depth and further scrutinize its productive effects within the apparatuses of neuroliberal governance examined throughout this book.

After repeated comments about his well-being on the Feed, I asked Aron if the term *digital well-being* meant anything to him. He replied, "I've never really thought of it as 'digital well-being.' It's just all, as they say, under the same branch for me because it's such an everyday part of our lives. It's not something I see as separate." I asked Geoff the same question after he detailed his own struggles with the Feed. Geoff was slow in his response: "Digital well-being. That's a really good question. The reason I'm pausing for thought is because—because so much of our lives are digital nowadays and we do so many things on the web, where does your digital well-being start, and your actual well-being and your mental well-being begin?" Instead, users spoke about managing the digital aspects of their lives as part of the balance of well-being. When asked to describe what well-being meant to her, Mia replied: "I think the word that kind of comes to mind is *balance*, because I think everything is okay when it's balanced. Like physical, mental, emotional, spiritual well-being—having that beautiful balance of health through all of them." Sharon, in a response that revealed her background in social work and psychology, replied: "So, for me, well-being is a sense of dynamic equilibrium, where life is moving forward, but it's nicely balanced. You need good health, good relationships, and of course you've got your Maslow's hierarchy of needs that need to be met, like food, shelter, water, housing, sanitation, all those basic things. But well-being for me is space, privacy, countryside, really good friends, lovely family, dignity, and integrity, and being healthy." Franny, a graphic designer in her early twenties, replied:

> I guess I would say it's everything in kind of proportion, so don't overdo it with one thing. So, I mean, obviously well-being, we all know that exercise is good for you, but then too much of that can have a negative effect. I'd say everything in moderation would be

what well-being is. I mean, people go on these crazy diets, but then that's never good for you in the long term, so, again, have that cake, but just don't have it every day. So, I'd say well-being for me would be a little bit of everything but in moderation.

Finally, Lucas simply replied that, for him, well-being meant "peace of mind, balance, not feeling stressed." As we can see, the responses of participants contradict the atomized presentation of self-interested social well-being found in Facebook's own vision of the digital good life, discussed at length in chapter 1. Instead, living well online, for these users, was not separate from living well offline, and could in no way be reduced to the accretion of neoliberally conceived credits of social capital, as Facebook would have us believe.

For some users, achieving the balance of well-being was predicated on acknowledging and cultivating the things in their life that provided peace and contentment, while guarding against those triggers or behaviors that led to feelings of unwellness, however that was understood. For Tobi, well-being constitutes "having an understanding of what causes you certain emotions and understanding what will make you feel a certain way, in order to not feel trapped by emotions . . . to know where not to go if you really don't want to feel a certain way, so you're kind of aware of how your lifestyle and how your decisions have consequences for you." Hanna expressed similar thoughts about knowing what impacts your mood on a personal level:

> Well-being I guess would be living life in a way that impacts positively, and I guess that differs for different people. . . . I guess for me I'm very involved in exercise. I find that very healthy. It makes me very happy. For other people it wouldn't be so much. Maybe they're involved in creative things, music, that sort of stuff. It's a way of living that maximizes your mental happiness, and that will differ with different people.

During the interviews, users all had a coherent sense of what was supposed to be good for them on the Feed. Controlled use, conscious engagements, attentive intention—the hallmarks of digital self-control explored at length throughout this book. Accordingly, these expressions of balance on the Feed guided users' conduct insofar as they advocate for and warn against particular styles of social media practice. The way users determined what scrolling relations need to be balanced, and how, can be revelatory of what Rahel Jaeggi terms *forms of life* on the Feed—implicitly normative cultural ensembles that function through the problematization, and solution, of human practices.[37] Specifically, we should note that these practices were all viewed as a personal responsibility to balance their well-being on social media. As such, and to repeat the point that this chapter has been making all along, users inhabited the role of the responsibilized user of Facebook and performed the neuroliberal nudges of self-control found therein, despite not recognizing the associated terms of discretized digital well-being. This self-positioning, and conceptual ambiguities, often carried a heavy burden, as we'll see below.

The Functions of Shame and Guilt

As already indicated, the interviewees described their struggles with the Feed through moralized idioms of distress associated with blame, shame, and guilt.[38] Even though all offered well-articulated rationales for why they were struggling to contain their interactions with the Feed—particularly through sophisticated critiques of the erstwhile social media attention economy and its corresponding forms of persuasive design—participants nevertheless spoke about their use as if (1) it was problematic and (2) its being so was principally their own fault. Existing research has demonstrated how users often feel pressure to live up to the demands for connection on social media.[39] Interestingly, the participants felt guilty about not being able to control their interactions with the Feed in a balanced manner, as if adopting these behaviors was something they had the capacity to control in the first place—a finding that supports other recent work in the field of disconnection studies.[40] This finding also resonates with some descriptions of guilt as resulting from negative "attributions referring to controllable and specific aspects of the self," revealing that users were, indeed, internalizing the discourses of user autonomy peddled by interested actors, such as social media companies.[41] This view, as explored at length in this book, positions self-controlled use as the chief correlate to feelings of positive individual well-being on social media. What is more, corresponding expressions of shame, which more closely relate to the public observability of perceived personal failures, and the negative attributions that come with that, further hint at the existence of an operative shared expectation of healthy use, which the watching eyes of each individual social network were imagined to be witnessing, assessing, and judging.[42] Here, the inability to control healthy habits on the Feed was deemed a personal failure on a public stage, guilt-inducing and shameful in equal measure.

The idioms of scrolling distress described by users throughout the interviews are understandable, considering the mediatized mixed messaging surrounding social media well-being that were circulating in the UK at the time. On one hand, individuals were being encouraged to get busy on the Feed, communicate for the sake of their own social success and well-being, and brand themselves as active, popular users in the eyes of their social network. This view is endorsed by media giants like Facebook, which have an interest in maintaining such active (profitable) use of their services. On the other hand, users were being told that they needed to resist the Feed's attentive pull, maintain distance from social media conventions, and balance their use as part of broader regimes of self-care—as expressed in popular self-help discourses of healthy technological relations. Participants' use of idioms of distress that expressed confusion, vice, shame, and guilt are therefore hardly surprising. Yet, rather than being a bug, these contradictions, and the uncertainty they foster, should be understood as a key feature of the psycho-computational discourses of time well spent and healthy social media use explored in this book so far. The ways in which users refer to the types of behavioral changes encouraged by governments, platforms, and NGOs indicate the presence of a hegemonic moral economy of ideal healthy social media use, a *structure of feeling* perhaps, that entrenches the dominant neuroliberal tropes extant within the UK of their interviews. The participants were keen to express awareness of this regime while scrolling down the Feed, and often positioned themselves as personally responsible for their imagined failure to overcome the attentive demands placed on them by Facebook. Consequently, some of these users felt compelled enough to confess their imagined failures to me as we scrolled, as demonstrated in the related discourses of personal responsibility we have encountered so far.

For example, Nadia described Facebook as "the shameful" platform, illustrating a sentiment expressed by almost all of the participants during the interviews. Nadia claimed she regularly felt like "you shouldn't be using" Facebook and spoke about her "constant battle of feeling like I'm addicted to using it and the shame of that." Nadia said her wish to leave Facebook was motivated by corresponding desire to feel "superior to other people because you've managed to come off [it]." When asked to expand on these feelings, and how they were encountered on the Feed, Nadia referred to the prevalence of posts from wellness influencers that encouraged practices of digital disconnection. She described the moralizing impact of these posts as we scrolled down her Feed:

A post will come up that is like "Stop scrolling! Instead, take a breath with me," and things like that. I've even considered doing a post like that of my own. So, I get it. It's supposed to be helpful, so people are putting those posts up to say, "Hey, stop scrolling, take a breath, be a bit more mindful," and that's good. But at the same time there's that inherent shame of like, "Oh crap, here I wasn't being mindful, I was just scrolling!" So yeah, the shame of using it comes from using it.

Ana Jorge has revealed the way these types of wellness influencer posts serve to buttress the very forms of capitalist value extraction from social media they seek to critique, a modality of (non)use that Laura Portwood-Stacer instructively refers to as *performative media refusal*.[43] From Nadia's comments, however, we can also see how such performances concurrently inculcate experiences of shame for those who come across them on their Feeds.

During her interview, Elsie spoke about her career concerns, her precarious hourly job as a waitress, and the worries this brought her. For Elsie, scrolling through Facebook felt like procrastination, taking her away from her search for a more secure job. She spoke of the "guilt" that came with scrolling inattentively on the Feed, describing it as a "waste of time." When asked to expand on her comment, Elsie said:

> So, I think it's that idea that I always have to be doing something "productive" that's going to, like, extend my knowledge or enhance my skills [or] achieve things that I think that I need. . . . Yeah, I think it's this inherited idea that I waste time a lot. For example, I think if I could choose the thing that I wouldn't have to pressure myself into doing, it would just be, like, laying in bed watching TV. I think I see that as a waste because I don't think I'm—I don't feel like I'm growing or I'm learning.

Later in the interview, Elsie related her struggles to control her scrolling activity and the guilt this led to in terms of a "neoliberal" vision of well-being:

Like when I think of well-being, the first thing that comes to mind is this very neoliberal idea of well-being that is constantly pushed on us. And it [conscious scrolling] is another thing to do. It's like you *have* to do it. Follow this exercise app and do your twenty minutes a day, and then eat this thing, engage with this thing, do your self-care. It's very individualized and it's very—it's just an extra added stress in my life generally.

Hence, managing time on social media so that it is *well spent* constituted yet another source of stress for Elsie, in an already pressurized situation. However, the strain of being productive was also felt by Bobby, in his sixties and employed full time, who said that scrolling for too long makes him "feel quite guilty." Despite these two contrasting economic situations, Bobby felt that scrolling down the Feed likewise forced him to question, "Why haven't I done something more productive with that time, rather than wasting it?"

Judy Wacjman has demonstrated how expressions of time pressure are inextricably bound to the sociotechnical hopes and fears of the day, as they specifically relate to the emergence of particular technologies.[44] Here, we can see how the Feed represents a site of concern for users who are worried about how they are spending their time productively in digital realms. As Elsie insightfully revealed, however, these discourses of productivity do not begin and end with the Feed. Elsie pinpointed her feelings of distress to operative neoliberal discourses that enjoin individuals to envisage themselves as bundles of self-cultivated, valuable skills that can be traded in an equal labor market. This imagines that humans are valuable only insofar as they are improving their skills, making the most of their time to do so, and actively differentiating their abilities against other competitors through comparable processes of self-improvement. This very much relates to the discourses of social capital as well-being explored in chapter 1, whereby Facebook's users are encouraged to view their relationships as resources to further self-interested goals in an open network, and their lives as ventures of ever-expanding personal development. As human productivity is imagined to be restricted by nothing other than individual application and psychological motivation, failing to be productive by not spending time wisely on the Feed represents a personal failure on the part of the individual. Accordingly, it follows that any personal feelings of guilt for this failure are completely warranted.

The Psychic Costs of Responsibilization

Through the various idioms of distress that users employed to describe their interactions with the Feed, we can begin to observe the psychic costs of responsibilization—costs incurred by adopting the neuroliberal vision of self-controlled active use as the key to social media well-being in the present day. It is not only the content and extractive design of the Feed environment that users perceive as troubling, but their own perceived (in)ability to inhabit this environment in a controlled, healthy, manner. The idioms of distress related to overwhelm, depression, anxiety, guilt, and shame that were expressed by these users indicate that these failings were primarily imagined to be the user's fault, and the user's fault alone. To reiterate a core argument that this book has been making throughout, such descriptions of individualized blame work to sever productive analytic links that could be made between these personal feelings of digital distress, and the broader economic, political, and cultural apparatuses of power that such feelings are cradled within, and to which they respond to and relate.

Let us return to Tobi's story to draw out the consequences of this severance. Tobi was unemployed at the time of his interview. He described how the Feed prompted him to compare his state of unemployment to the lives of other, more financially secure users in his network. This caused him anxiety and low self-esteem. If we were to give Tobi advice through the dominant lenses of atomized habits and self-controlled use explored in this book, our guidance would be to encourage Tobi to manage the time he spends on social media each day so that he can avoid encountering these presentations. The Feed getting you down, Tobi? Simply control how long you spend scrolling! Limit your use, buddy. While glib, such advice gives us reasons to pause for thought. Will advising Tobi to manage the time he spends scrolling through his Feed sufficiently assuage his anxieties of unemployment? And what will this do to how we understand the specific issues that Tobi is facing in his daily life? In Tobi's case, focusing solely on controlling his social media habits as the key correlate to his well-being online does not address the structural factors that contribute to his experience of unemployment, or why they are deemed shameful. This lack of questioning implicitly accepts the cultural disparagement of those who find themselves out of work, whether by choice or not. In ignoring these considerations, and simply telling Tobi to get a grip on his digital habits for the sake of his own health, we seem to be saying to him: yes, being unemployed is something to be inherently worried about; yes, it is your fault; and yes, it is best to avoid anything that reminds you of these facts. Rather than confront the logic behind these assertions, or question where they come from and how they are presently enforced, then, the advice to simply avoid reminders of them by avoiding the Feed simply reinforces their saliency. Ignorance through topical exclusion, that is, reinstates and reasserts their imagined truth. Put another way, to refuse to examine the contextual factors that contribute to specific and qualitatively unique feelings of distress online is to legitimize the styles of shame, guilt, and blame expressed by users like Tobi. This implicitly validates the forces they respond to as a result.

If you are instead concerned with reducing these felt pressures, and would like to offer users like Tobi, and perhaps yourself, a way to rethink feelings of digital distress on social media, other interpretive lenses are available. Chiefly, perhaps we could begin by recognizing the arbitrariness of these pressures and position them within the networks of power through which they derive their force. Here we could hold in stasis these ideas, destabilizing their momentum in doing so, rather than endorsing their efficacy. Returning to Tobi's case, since when was not being productive such a bad thing? And why is being out of work such a source of shame? This is in no way to deny the feeling of these ties—which, as we can see from the interview data above, are all too real—but is instead to emphasize the need to critique the specific cultural ensembles of power that hold them fast. I argue that we should focus on how this power is materially expressed and channeled through technologies like social media, which have no real interest in seeing their force diminished. Guilt, that is, functions as yet another affective bond that maintains users' profitable interactive presence on the Feed. We ought to recognize how social media like Facebook explicitly profits off this personal shame and guilt, as it does with concurrent feelings of joy, connection, hope, anxiety, depression, and the rest. This analytic opening allows us to fully face up to the ambivalent force of social media and has the potential to lead to new vocabularies of change as a result.

The idioms of distress expressed above, if nothing else, show how responsibilized discourses are failing users. Following the thought of critical theorist Nancy Fraser, we cannot dismiss "people's intuitions about what is and isn't 'working' as if they were fundamentally mistaken in some way."[45] Rather, Fraser continues, "we should be trying to clarify those intuitions" in order to better distinguish their qualities and examine their effects.[46] For Fraser, "this requires theorizing from a standpoint that is sensitive to the experience of capitalism's subjects, which is already laden with social interpretations and normative evaluations. We want to understand the sources of these interpretations and evaluations, whether and how they can be justified, and how to understand disagreements over them."[47] The role of the researcher, or the intellectual if you'd like, is to work backward from the intuitions, perceptions, and experiences of everyday people in order to situate our calls for change directly in response to them. Such a stance relates to the call by Raymond Williams, himself working with the thought of Gramsci, to position intellectual work as part of a broader political process, one that is able to illuminate current epistemological limits and why they ought to be challenged.[48] By looking beyond taken-for-granted discourses of digital self-control, and in pointing out their economic and normalizing function, I hope to have shown how critical research can help users better understand their personal intuitions of social media guilt and shame, with the hope that doing so could lead to new targets of their chagrin and critique. Might we do better to see where the feelings of shame, guilt, and blame on the Feed come from, and distinguish them from the individual subject carrying them? Could we ask why such feelings seem to impact some users more than others, and whether we can offer ways to understand the situation with less judgment and more empathy? And are there ways for users to further distance themselves from the techniques they are offered to understand and act upon their personal experiences of digital distress, and form new ones in response? The conclusion of this book will now face these questions head on.

Conclusion

A Different Ethics of Living Well Online

So far, this book has employed Foucauldian analytics to examine the normative relations generated through discourses, designs, and habits of social media well-being. Along with its methodological grounding in sociotechnical script analysis, empirical focus on neuroliberal responsibilization, and angles of inquiry inspired by disconnection studies and cultural studies, the preceding chapters have been gathered roughly along the lines of what Foucault described as three axes of analysis: the axis of knowledge, the axis of power, and the axis of ethics.[1] As has hopefully become clear to the reader by now, these axes triangulate and are self-supporting, through both their consistencies and contradictions. First, the axis of knowledge, following Foucault, is concerned with the question of how humans are constituted as subjects of knowledge—how they are known, positively or negatively, how they are measured, tracked, compared, and, in some instances, set against each other. Chapter 1 revealed how healthy users of social media are scripted as self-interested subjects in Facebook's psychological research and public relations materials. We saw how these users were imagined to be impelled to connect with their social ties on platforms to fulfill their supposedly innate needs of evolutionary human belonging. Healthy active social media use, in this framework, is presented as a normal expression of human life and, upon this basis, provides users a naturalized reason to practice active (profitable) engagement with platforms. This is despite the apparent psychological risks posed by engaging with social media in any way at all. We observed the way users of social media are made intelligible through intermingled rubrics of neoliberal social capital, evolutionary teleological discourses, psycho-computational modes of measurement, and tool-views of technology. I argued that it is through these intersecting dimensions that Facebook's healthy users are made known and visible as beings of a certain type.

Chapter 2 explored internal inconsistencies within this grid of intelligibility, revealed when examining how Facebook statedly designs for user well-being on the platform. This insight emerged through an engagement with the second of Foucault's analytics, the axis of power, which is concerned with how humans are "constituted as subjects who exercise or submit to power relations."[2] Specifically, we saw how the design of Facebook's user interfaces, such as the Feed, function to prompt modes of active use. This was used to evidence Facebook's implicit distrust in the capacity of users to act in their own "rational" well-being interests on the platform. A core dilemma emerged here: If users were actually predisposed to actively use social media, why would they need to be encouraged to do so through technical nudges? This disconnect was the basis for my argument that the forms of healthy active social media use currently presented to us are not as natural, and thus not as inevitable, as many would have us believe. Instead, I argued that the modes of digital wellness technically and discursively administered by social media companies like Facebook are better understood as attempts to conduct the conduct of users toward a range of activity that secures platforms' continued datafied capitalist functioning. Chapter 2 thus examined the constitution of users as technically governable subjects for particular strategic purposes.

Chapter 3 analyzed data created through interviews with British Facebook users to see how users themselves were responding to the material discursive scripting of healthy use in their everyday lives. We saw how the individualized, responsibilized, and neuroliberal targeting of habit as the key correlate of social media well-being was reflected in users' expressions of guilt and shame when describing their personal failure to control their own digital habits. This chapter was oriented around the third of Foucault's axes of analysis, the axis of ethics, which questions how humans are "constituted as moral subjects of [their] own actions."[3] Rather than their diminished feelings of well-being on social media offering an entry point for discussing the relations of power involved in their activation, we instead witnessed how users' psychic distress online was mainly turned inward, nullifying social media well-being as a potential site of political intervention, and increasing the unfair pressures felt by users to live well in a (digital) world that is perhaps not set up for them to do so as they wish. Foucault once questioned "how light power would be, and easy to dismantle no doubt, if all it did was to observe, spy, detect, prohibit and punish."[4] Chapter 3 instead revealed how power "incites, provokes, produces" forms of life, modes of expression, and styles of conduct for people to adopt and live by.[5] This is evident through the idioms of distress, guilt, and shame expressed by the users interviewed, as well as in the behaviors and self-nudges users put in practice to assuage them in response. Accordingly, the functioning of power examined in chapter 3, and throughout this book, "is not simply eye and ear," but something that has been shown to "make people act and speak."[6]

When combined, the three axes of analysis upon which this book turns reveal "the different modes by which, in our culture, human beings are made subjects," drawing attention to the particular styles of healthy living this opens up on social media, and those that it restricts.[7] At this stage, you may be thinking that all of this paints a fairly bleak picture: a tangled knot of responsibilized digital wellness, neuroliberal behaviorism, problematics of neoliberal freedom, topical exclusions of the social determinants of health, and datafied regimes of capitalist value-extraction. A tight bind, and one ironically secured by the free actions of individual users themselves—users who are simply trying to navigate the infiltration, psychological demands, and constitutive effects of social media in their daily lives. Yet, however grim, this situation is not irretrievable. A key argument that this book has been developing throughout is that apparatuses of governance can only be imagined otherwise if we have a lucid account of their current strategic functions. In highlighting these strategic functions, I hope to have fragmented what may have once been considered stable about social media well-being, while pointing toward fruitful lines of advancement in their wake.

This book, by revealing the contingencies, arbitrary points of articulation, and discursive material buttresses of social media well-being, has engaged, following Paul Rabinow, the practice of thinking as "an act of modal transformation from the constative to the subjunctive," from "the singular to the multiple."[8] In this conclusion, I want to more deeply explore the type of change that engaging with such multiple interpretations can motivate. To be clear, this will not be change based on their crude instrumentalization. This book's findings will not be used as a means to furnish *the* guide to the digital good life, or to establish *the* healthy habits for beleaguered users to adopt in response to the stated toxicity of platforms. Rather, I want to see how the Foucauldian style of critique I have employed throughout this book can be used as the basis for alternative critical social media well-being interventions in the future—interventions that have decidedly indeterminate, open ends.

Below, I will present an "attitude, an ethos, a philosophical life" that provides individuals an opportunity to refuse what has been granted to them in the discourses, designs, and habits of individualized social media well-being to date.[9] We will explore what chance we have to refuse our constructions as (ir)rational creatures of self-interest in technologized spheres, and how this could provide an opening to refuse the means through which we have been led to understand our strengths and flaws in neuroliberal systems of governance. Foucault calls this effort the "critical ontology of ourselves," the "analysis of the limits imposed on us and an experiment with the possibility of going beyond them."[10] Although this approach is purposefully unsettling and, as we will see, carries significant ontological risks, the discomfort it could cause should not mistakenly be dismissed as a nihilistic indulgence, or as a peculiar form of "moral dandyism."[11] Instead, I will argue that it is precisely within these breakages, within these risks, that the very possibility (if not naive hope) for new modes of living well with social media can be found, however slim, and however unlikely it may presently seem.

The Limit Attitude

The term Foucault gives to this approach is the *limit attitude*, often also described as the *historico-critical attitude*.[12] These terms are somewhat interchangeable, insofar as they both establish a critical orientation toward the present day based on (1) the problematization of current epistemic conditions and an examination of where they derive their force, (2) a testing of the forms of conduct associated with these conditions, and (3) an ethical exploration of what life is and could be within and without them. In this way, the limit attitude triangulates the three axes of analysis discussed above, encompassing a general "critique of what we are saying, thinking, and doing" in contemporary locales.[13] In this stance toward the present moment, the Foucauldian style of critique echoes Enlightenment concerns with contemporaneity and its questioning of tradition and accepted forms of knowledge. In particular, Foucault establishes resonances between his thought and Kant's diagnostics of cosmopolitanism, taking the latter's call to *dare to know* as a key moment in the development of a distinctly Western style of self-aware criticism.[14] With Kant, a Prussian philosopher writing in the mid- to late eighteenth century, critical thinking became an overtly liberatory practice for the first time. Specifically, the critique in Kant's anthropological and journalistic writings is imbued with a force to propel humanity toward a freer future grounded on reason and proper legal constraints.[15]

In particular, examining and overcoming the current barriers to reason, for Kant, was a form of intellectual ground clearing—paving the way for a rational world-historical system to emerge in its wake. However, while the general disposition toward freedom is shared, the limit attitude encouraged by Foucault is distinct from Kant's in two significant ways. First, Kantian critique sought to uncover innate human traits in order to formalize a path toward universal values, political frameworks, and social structures.[16] Foucauldian critique, on the other hand, aims to introduce discontinuity into precisely these "natural" forms of human life and organization. Second, and relatedly, this means that the cosmopolitan state toward which Kant's critique strives plays no such leading role in the adoption of the limit attitude for Foucault. Rather than critique being put into the service of a teleological destination, whatever that may be, the future that Foucauldian critique opens is unknown from the outset.

Much as with governance, the very efficacy of the limit attitude is predicated on the existence of free subjects, with the ability to first identify, give shape to, and then act in accordance with their own beliefs and desires. Foucault's free subjects are individuals who can give themselves "the right to question truth," imagine alternative courses of action if necessary, and explore the potential to exist differently in the world in response.[17] For Thomas Lemke, accordingly, the limit attitude is characterized by three interrelated aspects: "the activity of problematization, the art of voluntary insubordination, and the audacity to expose one's own status as a subject."[18] Foucault describes the limit attitude in terms of *experience*, a dynamic and risky interplay of these games of truth, forms of power, and ethical relations to the self.[19] Critique can be understood, therefore, as a form of analytic distancing, a stepping back from accepted ordinances.

This distancing does not suggest an outside perspective, as if to verify the existence of a stable viewpoint able to objectify human experience once and for all. No, what Foucault is instead pointing toward is "a historical ontology of ourselves," where we, *you*, the individual, are both the subject and object of analysis, both the subject and object of critique.[20] Foucault is asking us to make strange what may have otherwise appeared familiar, and to extricate ourselves from the neat historical and cultural lineages that grant a sense of normalcy to current ways of doing things. Further to this, like his teacher Georges Canguilhem, Foucault takes the notion of normality as a point of departure. Basic questions follow. How is this mode of life normal to me, at this moment in time? How have I learned the habits that constitute it? From whom? From where? And when? Simply understood, such questions aim to help individuals more firmly situate themselves within their present, without having to rely only on the common, maybe dominant, narratives available to them within their own milieus to do so. Such narratives, as this book has explored throughout, like all narratives, purport their own histories, values, and epistemic thresholds. Rather than accept traditional rationales for the way things are, for the way *you are*, the limit attitude instead asks the individual to question the contingent chances that have coalesced to form their own stable image of contemporaneity, as well as the stories they have been told to explain its current appearance.

Introducing discontinuity into the scene of the present may seem like a needless intervention if you sit comfortably within its confines. Yet not having to question one's own experience in the world is a hallmark of privilege. Foucault is encouraging the individual to step outside the entrenched associations of personhood that they have been previously offered, regardless of whether they have ever felt the need to do so before. One consequence of the limit attitude is to bring the disparities between its felt necessity into relief. Why haven't I felt impelled to question myself before? Why do I feel as if it is all I do? For some, the reassuring stability of the self will vanish. For others, its void will be given a clearer shape.

Importantly, and foregrounding something I will return to later on, the self for Foucault does not describe a single, separate, immutable thing, but rather a process of self-relation. For Foucault, the self emerges—is formed, as it were—in the activities "whereby the subject reflexively relates to itself."[21] Posing the type of questions above is one way to engage this process of self-relation, helping the individual to more clearly assess the accepted means of becoming a valuable subject that are available to them in the present day, and those practices they have been led to avoid. In the context of this book, we can recall the way active social media use promises the individual a chance to become a productive healthy subject, while passive scrolling and bad habits online lead to their denigration. It is precisely these self-relations that have been under scrutiny throughout.

As Louisa Cadman writes, the limit attitude "presupposes a subject who questions, but it also supposes that the subject is simultaneously de-subjugated through the very act of questioning. In simple terms, to bring forth and question a field of subjection means that the subject cannot be quite what it was before."[22] Because of this, the critical ontology of ourselves is a risky business. Refusing the comfort of contemporarily apparent forms of subjectivation pulls the rug from under the individual. Judith Butler writes that "to criticize," with Foucault, "means to expose one's own ontological status," which necessarily "involves the danger of falling outside the established norms of recognition."[23] This risk has been too great for some to bear in the past. Without historical norms, for example, how can political communities commit to shared values?[24] What are the criteria of judgment that lead to collective improvements?[25] And does all of this simply end up creating an individualistic mess of self-fashioned subjects, with confused moralities and clashing norms?[26] Maybe. But this somewhat misses the point. As Butler continues, Foucault is grasping toward something far more primary, a consideration of "who will be subject here, and what will count as life."[27] This is not to say that new norms, communities, and ethics cannot form through a collective engagement with the limit attitude—far from it, in fact. Rather, following Nietzsche, Foucault wants us to reconsider current epistemes that preconfigure what good and bad human practices are, and look beyond taken-for-granted accounts of how collective human communities are said to naturally grow.[28] Even more than this, as Butler points out, Foucault is ultimately challenging us to consider whether we are "willing, in the name of the human, to allow the human to become something other than what it is traditionally assumed to be."[29]

Counter-conduct, Care of the Self

In this book, I have been working with an understanding of governance as the "modes of action, more or less considered and calculated, which [are] destined to act upon the possibilities of action of other people."[30] Through this, I have shown how widely available discourses and designs of healthy social media use establish a "possible field of action" within which individual users are led to consider, act upon, and relate to their own well-being.[31] Specifically, this is well-being imagined as a responsibilized endeavor of controlled active use. This book has shown how the conduct of conduct mobilized through the governance of social media well-being operates through regimes of psycho-computational power/knowledge/topical exclusions (chapter 1); technical nudges built into the design of platforms (chapter 2); and the thoughts, activities, and reflections of users themselves (chapter 3). By explicating the contingencies upon which all of this is built, it has been my intention to disturb the ease with which dominant visions of social media well-being are presently accepted. Throughout, I hope to have shown how refusing the current logics, techniques, and instruments of social media well-being opens the opportunity to not be governed "like that, by that, in the name of those principles, [and] with such and such an objective in mind."[32] In the following, I will focus on *counter-conduct* and *care of the self* as two related tactics that can contribute to this effort.[33]

As I have already mentioned, freedom for Foucault is "the condition for the exercise of power" and is at the "same time its precondition."[34] Exercises of power, then, always have "the possibility of recalcitrance" produced through them.[35] Because of this, conduct and the possibility to be otherwise are always under question in analytics of governance—something Olga Demetriou recognizes as a distinctly "political dynamic."[36] As Ben Golder clarifies: "Within any form of conduct . . . there is the immanent possibility of a counter-conduct—of something which resists, works against, subverts, or avoids the operation of the attempt to govern conduct, . . . [and] this possibility is disclosed by the workings of government itself. Where there is power, there is resistance."[37] Counter-conducts, writes Arnold Davidson, "are movements characterised by wanting to be conducted differently" and "whose objective is a different type of conduction."[38] Bringing forth a counter-conduct through intellectual work is to "indicate an area in which each individual can conduct" themselves differently, in thought and behavior.[39] Criticisms of governance, as such, are always immanent to the terrain of governance that is put under scrutiny. The critic is at once the vehicle and target of critique. While this position *within* governance is always a compromised existence, it is precisely this situation that renders the critic attentive to "possible flights" from its workings.[40]

In this book, I have shown how such a stance can allow governed users to hold in stasis the masquerading benevolence of social media's discursive and material well-being interventions. Alternatively rendered as part of a strategic field of conduct, the user may instead wish to look more closely at the attempted naturalization of healthy, active social media use. How am I being led to situate myself in these domains? What constitutes "normal" activity for me to adopt here? And where are these ideas coming from? Some may be content with the answers they find. Others won't be. For the latter, further questions can follow. What effects are incurred through adopting these subject-positions? What present possibilities do they hold in place? What futures do they block? The preceding chapters have offered my own partial responses to these types of questions. But it is the style of questioning itself that is important. Insofar as the limit attitude can help individuals more thoroughly situate themselves within normative relations of power, a more precise account of their felt pressures and discomforts can be discerned.

Foucault invites us to consider these questions, these forms of self-relation, in terms of *care of the self*—the "methods and techniques" by which the self makes itself an "object to be known" in different ways.[41] This self-positioning, for Foucault, can expose lines of flights for the self to explore, new ways to differently constitute the self as a self. As I have already mentioned, this can only happen because the self is not something that is considered preformed or fixed. Rather, the self can be understood as an active process of self-relating—between the self and the self, the self and the world, and the self and others. As Daniel W. Smith puts it, "We must understand the two principles—'care' and 'self'—not as two independent substances interacting with one another, but rather as inherently interrelated concepts, which always operate on the same plane."[42] The self in care of the self, as such, operates in both the "objective and subjective genitive" senses: "that which does the caring" while also "the object of that same care."[43]

Foucault examined the possibilities and constraints of care of the self through an engagement with ancient Greco-Roman ethics, specifically regarding how the ancients established appropriate forms of conduct in public life.[44] As opposed to the individual being free to be whatever they wish, the self-cultivation that comes with care of the self instead is necessarily formed in relation to the world that surrounds us—with the allowances and frictions it provides different individuals, at different times. As Diana Stypinska puts it, this involves "a constantly evolving relation to ourselves, others, and the world," and is something that "we actively maintain throughout our lives."[45] The specific means that individuals have available for them to do so change over time and are dependent on the historical and cultural environment of their existence. For instance, examples of generating self-knowledge from the ancients include writing, journaling, meditation, thought experiments, and self-examinations.[46] Foucault calls these means "practices of self," whereby subjects mold themselves in an "active fashion."[47]

Such practices of self, however, are not "something that the individual invents" alone.[48] Rather, "they are patterns that he finds in his culture and which are proposed, suggested and imposed on him by his culture, his society and his social group."[49] This is the world of norms we have been examining throughout this book: social mores, traditions, and their disruptions, the contested habits of thought and behavior that condition the existence of individuals at certain times and places. From the preceding chapters, think of the way healthy social media users are led to cultivate themselves as beings of a certain type through active use of platforms, and how this carries with it a decidedly moralized purpose. Think back to the ways in which active use is promised to users both as the path toward their natural belonging on platforms and, contrastingly, as a means to overcome their natural fallibilities. And consider how the digital good life is promised to users if they would only control their social media activity in a conscious way. These practices are presented to users as fixed. Unchangeable. Soundly reasoned. Yet if the care of the self indicates that there are innumerable ways for the self to be constituted, its attempted fixing through the arbitrary contemporary practices of healthy active use on social media ought to raise a few eyebrows.

I have shown how such practices, rather than being a natural extension of normal human life, tie users to the neoliberal, capitalist, and behaviorist milieu within which they are expressed. The means of self-relation they offer users are thus constrained by these conditions. We are asked to relate to our friends and loved ones on social media as resources, valuable to us only insofar as they can help us accrue social capital in the future. We are asked to relate to ourselves as fallible, indolent subjects, easily distracted by the attentive demands of platforms. We are asked to relate to the world as if we were solely responsible for the habits we choose in response to these demands, and personally culpable if our well-being suffers through our inability to control our actions. We are asked to trade all our hopes and struggles online for personal data, for the sake of platforms' profits. Now, considering the many potential shapes of the self that Foucault shows are available to us, I would contend that these practices, the subjects they produce, and the ideas and interests that motivate them offer a sadly diminished account of what humans could be. I have argued that by holding all of this in stasis, we can more clearly question whether they are forms we wish to inhabit for ourselves, now and in the future.

Such questions, which point toward something fundamental in our lives, are, for Foucault, a way to ascertain and act upon truth in the tangled terrains of power/knowledge within which we live. Indeed, we could consider the exploration of and answers to these questions a form of truth-telling, something Foucault examines as *parrēsia*.[50] This term describes how speakers render truths about their own lives in the world, to themselves and others, as "manifest, present, perceptible, and active."[51] This is not the revealing of truth as simple "transmission," but the *telling* of truth in order for the individual "to challenge and change oneself; to disrupt the trajectory of their private orbit and to attain a different mode of being."[52] The *parrhesiast*, according to Dana Villa, is someone involved in a "struggle against endlessly proliferating (and resurrected) illusions," someone who seeks new interpretations that can disturb hegemonic beliefs, and someone who takes risks in "frank and fearless" speech to do so.[53] Because of this, parrēsia has been examined as a discursive mode that facilitated the development of practical, democratic reason in Hellenistic antiquity, in the fourth and fifth centuries in particular, whereby counsel to power could be heard and acted upon.[54]

Accordingly, Foucault suggests that the "most important part of the parrhesiastic function" is to "point out to the subject" their "place in the world," whether that is to themselves, their peers, or those in positions of authority.[55] Upon this basis, the parrhesiast is "someone who has to say things about what man is in general, about the order of the world, and about the necessity of things."[56] In establishing this, parrēsia, as Boris Traue points out, "interrupts habits or beliefs entertained about oneself," opening space for new ways of being to emerge in response.[57] As such, the type of truth telling involved in care of the self is ultimately a "conversion of power," insofar as it produces self-generated configurations of power, knowledge, and truth, new perspectives on governance, and new modes of subjectivation for the individual to consider and act upon.[58] What once may have appeared controlling and limiting could, through these processes, become something more malleable and open to change.[59]

New Reflections on Healthy Use

In the case of social media well-being, pressured users are given an opportunity to rethink and reshape the demands placed upon them through practices associated with care of the self and the related practices of parrēsia. Now we will explore how this could work in actuality. What to do if the individual user finds that the clothes of the healthy user do not quite fit? If, despite best efforts, the discomfort caused by platforms is too great? If the extraction of value from their activity online is deemed too unfair? If the link to neoliberal responsibilization is too raw? If the nudge choice architectures feel too constraining? What then?

Bluntly, one option could be for disaffected users to simply quit social media. Despite the stated difficulty of this effort, as both the disconnection studies literature and the qualitative data explored in chapter 3 have shown, this line of flight remains quite clear. The counter-conduct of quitting, however, as with all counter-conducts, is not a totalizing solution to the problematics of governance at hand. Instead, quitting social media ought to be viewed as an event that can crack open the problem space in a new way, something that allows the individual to see its thresholds in a different light. Without social media, that is, the problem of social media well-being simply becomes the problem of well-being. Following this, the individual exposes a glaring and maybe irresolvable question at the heart of the matter: What is well-being? This is no easy confrontation. Yet without one of its potentially confounding technological elements in the equation, the individual (ex-user) can stage the scene in new ways. What shapes of well-being can I now try on? What fits me best? What other activities will fill the gap left by scrolling? What relationships can I foster beyond the narrow functionality of likes? And how will my other personal relationships with technology factor into this?

Quitting social media, obviously, may not be desirable for all. Some gain plenty of pleasure, social connection, and value from engaging with platforms. For those who struggle with social media but wish to persist, other counter-conducts may emerge from an engagement with care of the self and the parrhesiastic function. For instance, recognizing the very recent historical character of self-controlled active social media use, or any social media use at all for that matter, could be one way for the individual to release some of the felt pressure to conform to its current parameters. As previous chapters have shown, the norms of responsibilized healthy use are imbued with a distinctly neoliberal flavor, working through more recent developments of neuroliberal behavioral management. Making these links explicit could give individuals a chance to interpret the directives of healthy use with a more critical eye. When individuals feel encouraged to adopt practices of self-controlled use to manage their well-being online, as expressed by social media companies, technical nudges, governments, and well-meaning interlocutors, being able to identify the interlocking psychological, political, and computational logics employed to do so could enable a better assessment of whether they wish to adhere to them. Do such practices hold together when scrutinized? Do they actually work for me? Do I wish to perpetuate their political effects, for myself, for others?

Regarding the effects of this type of historicized self-relation, Foucault writes that "saying that we are much more recent than we believe is not a way of placing all the burden of our history on our shoulders. Rather, it puts within the range of work which we can do to and for ourselves, the greatest possible part of what is presented to us as inaccessible."[60] In different terms, the work at stake here could help develop a new type of critical digital literacy, whereby not only the informational, economic, and (anti)democratic operations of platforms are surfaced for users, but also their discursive materializations and relationships to power/knowledge.[61] Beyond the problems of the echo chamber or filter bubbles, or misinformation and polarization, we could encourage a broader, more essential consideration of how platforms seek to condition and constrain the very possibility of human thought and activity in the world today. Indeed, recalling Judith Butler, we might consider how platforms technically demarcate what it means to be a human existing in the world at all. This does not promise easy answers to the questions of social media well-being, but at least situates their asking on more realistic, more humble, more personally relevant, ground.

Through this process, individuals may begin to question whether their well-being online really boils down to their individual actions on platforms. As seen in previous chapters, well-being encompasses multitudinous factors, is culturally relative, and is measurable in multiple ways. Reflecting on their own experience from this position, users may begin to question their own orientations and feelings toward social media well-being through a wider lens. For example, when assessing the situations where social media is a positive, negative, or ambivalent force in their lives, the individual could look to their wider life circumstances as salient points of reference. What was happening in their various relationships at the time, perhaps, that could have impacted their online experience? What of their senses of community that set the social scene of their scrolling? Of their feelings of belonging in the world? Their material circumstances? Their identities? Their physical body? And so on and so forth. From this standpoint, the self-relating user, with all these contributing factors in mind, may suddenly perceive the idea that their well-being on social media is solely the result of "good" active habits as a little ridiculous. The importance individuals place on their activity on social media may be altered in response, maybe into something more manageable, and hopefully less conducive to the type of shame and guilt produced in its dominant responsibilized shape. We can thus see how ameliorating the pressure individuals place on their social media activity opens space for new types of self-understanding to emerge, prompting correspondingly different styles of action to form in response.

Along with this self-situation, the recognition that social media well-being is entangled with broader infrastructures of capitalist datafication could provide users with another entry point to consider the issue. Indeed, as numerous thinkers have pointed out, the extent to which the inequalities and exploitation necessary within capitalist societies are conducive to well-being is an open question.[62] Considering the extractive capitalist functioning of data platforms, users struggling with their well-being on social media may wonder whether the economic characteristics of platforms themselves are implicated in their experience, a space where the entirety of social activity is transformed into profitable data, rendered valuable only insofar as it is measurable, scalable, and saleable. Through this analytic prism, both the alienation and targeting of desire that comes from users' *prosumer* positions become valid sites of psychosocial concern, rather than simply a site of abstracted analysis.[63] Tactically, as a counter-conduct, being able to link depreciations of well-being on social media to the economic machinations and styles of psychological alienation endemic to capitalism is a way to collectivize what is necessarily an individual experience—the conditions of platforms themselves become something that can connect users' personal struggles with well-being.[64] This is social media well-being imbued with a political economic charge, becoming a valid location of critique in the process.

A Different Ethics of Living Well

Counter-conduct and the care of the self form a dynamic "that transforms one's relation to oneself and to others."[65] They are "active interventions" in the "domain of the ethical and political practices and forces that shape us."[66] Such movements produce new subject positions, what Stypinska describes as a "process of *othering*."[67] By radically questioning the ontological grounds upon which we are constituted, we are able to loosen the ties that bind us to "prevailing ways of being and thinking" in different discursive material environments.[68] On the surface, this may come across as a uniquely individualized effort—something that results in a disconnected amalgamation of isolated subjects cut off from the collective concerns, values, and demands of the community at large. This critique has been leveled at Foucault's thought before.[69] Some have even drawn links between Foucault's focus on self-relation and neoliberalism's championing of dogged individuality.[70] However, as I have already hinted at, a different picture emerges when you look more closely at Foucault's writings.

Rather than all of this self-questioning, self-situation, and self-critique simply leading toward the refinement of a narcissistic, aesthetic individual—a being that thinks and acts in ethical isolation from public life—such activity, for Foucault, has precisely the opposite goal. Care of the self in the Foucauldian sense has the intention of securing the very possibility for an ethical public life to form at all. In Foucault's later writings, acting as part of a community of others requires a thorough and deep consideration of the self if those bonds are both to last and work for everyone involved. Foucault argues that the care of the self comes before care of the community, as the relationship of the self to the self is ontologically prior to relations toward the community.[71] Because ethical communities can form only if the individuals they comprise are ethically secure in and of themselves, Foucault suggests that caring for the self is both prior to and a precondition of caring for others. To understand this further, and to consider how this might finally factor into the development of a new ethics of living well with social media, it is worth positioning this view against common ideations of self-care that the reader may have encountered in popular spheres before.

In 2014, Sara Ahmed, via Audre Lorde, wrote about self-care as a form of "warfare," a means for discriminated subjects to preserve themselves in a racialized capitalist system opposed to their very existence.[72] Ahmed positioned her argument against the then prevalent view of self-care as a mere self-indulgence, something that exposes the moral selfishness of those who dare take the time for themselves at the expense of other, more productive pursuits.[73] Ahmed showed how such a view limits the possibilities of life, fashioning a moral economy that favors economically valuable activity rather than unproductive indolence. For Ahmed, by contrast, the weaponized view of self-care "is not about one's own happiness," but about finding ways to survive in a hostile world.[74] Accordingly, through cultivating these existences, self-care can become a generative political endeavor, a form of refusal. Collectively, these refusals can bring marginalized individuals and communities together in common struggles.

Over a decade on, however, the ubiquity of self-care as a modality of neoliberalized wellness perhaps diminishes its latent political potential. When every day we encounter encouragements to practice and consume self-care from governments, employers, banks, insurance companies, social media providers, and the rest, it is hard to imagine how self-care could function as a fulcrum of resistance within the contemporary order of things.[75] In contrast to care of the self, which sees individuals deeply consider the power relations through which they are made and take ontological risks to tell uncomfortable truths about their situation, much of self-care in its contemporary form is about employing techniques that enable you to sidestep these difficult questions and simply accept your position in the world, whatever that may be.[76] No need for any of this intense self-relating—have a bath, practice mindfulness, do some yoga. Retreat from the world in a comforting bubble of your own making.

Neoliberalized self-care also simultaneously pulls in the opposite direction. Think here of the tropes of self-care as self-improvement, whereby working on the self, whether physically, mentally, culturally, or socially, is a means to secure well-being for the future. Consider favorable habits such as exercise, therapy, and eating well as forms of upskilling, a way to invest in your own human capital and get ahead of the competition in the wellness stakes. Individuals are encouraged to make active changes to their lifestyles, cut out unhealthy habits, and adopt healthy ones instead. Get up and go for a run in the morning, don't laze in bed. Practice active use of platforms, don't doom scroll. As previously explored, these activities broadly relate to the prevalence of healthism doctrines in consumerist societies, whereby bodies, psychological moods, and well-being are states to be managed and optimized, ongoing projects that are readily supported by services and products available on the market.[77] Self-care, then, in the present-day context, contradictorily encourages subjects to accept their position in the world while also encouraging them to improve it through active interventions in their own lifestyle habits.

In this way, popular visions of self-care are both withdrawn and active. The former position, which asks us to radically disengage from the sources of our stress, has been understood as an appropriation of religiously inflected ideas of nonattachment, as found in various Buddhist traditions, which see detachment from the self and worldly concern as a vital spiritual endeavor.[78] The latter position, on the other hand, which asks users to optimize their well-being through behavioral interventions, has been productively related to neoliberal responsibilization, whereby individuals ought to constantly invest in themselves to better their situation for their own good.[79] This strange mix, which pulls the individual toward both release and engagement, combines to obscure any meaningful consideration of the wider social, cultural, and political factors that may be contributing to the need for any self-care in the first place. As opposed to the necessity of self-care signaling that something may be wrong with the environments within which it is practiced, neoliberalized self-care encourages an inward view where striving for your own well-being is the only goal.

Much as with the discourses and designs of digital wellness that have been under scrutiny in this book, self-care has become something universally positive, strangely conflated with the good, whose presence can actually be used to verify the caring and empathetic nature of the actually hostile exploitative environments it is deemed necessary within, such as the workplace or, indeed, social media. We can usefully understand this attempted foreclosure as a mode of what the critical theorist Herbert Marcuse would call *co-optation*, the process through which capitalist forces turn critiques of their operations to their own advantage.[80] Specifically, co-optation involves actors hollowing out the foundations of any meaningful critiques made against systemic issues, turning them inside out, and situating them on new discursive grounds with new connotative terms.

Where neoliberalized self-care could variously result in a blinkered focus on self-improvement, or a radical dissociation with the world, care of the self is "a way of caring for others," offering a template for ontologically engaged self-knowledge while also demarcating the common bonds and limits that enable communities to establish ethical conducts to begin with.[81] Although some have positioned care of the self in direct opposition to the more overtly radical political operations established by thinkers such as Lorde and Ahmed, I argue that Foucault's thought can likewise be used to establish collective responses to the diminishing of well-being in contemporary apparatuses of capitalism, as particularly witnessed on social media.[82] This is because that care of the self, although "self-regarding," is "not selfish" and, in fact, constitutes the "necessary condition for remaining open and available to other."[83]

Foucault demonstrates how, in the Hellenistic version of care of the self, this was especially important for those in positions of authority, where the risk of tyrannical power could undermine any given legitimacy to make decisions on behalf of others. Beyond this, and in the present day, to know yourself is to be attentive to, and to situate yourself within, circumstantial relations of power. It involves degrees of respect. First, that you are worthy of care, and second that your situation deserves to be different if it is not working in your favor. Importantly, care of the self also opens this possibility for others. That is, exploring the pathways of change for yourself is to simultaneously grant the same opportunity to those around you. More than this, to be sensitive to the relations of power through which you are constituted is to be sensitive to the relations of power that constitute others as well. It is to try and be aware of the different ways in which power pressures different individuals existing within the same community, producing different subject positions, different allowances to enjoy, different restrictions to endure. Cultivating respectful relations to yourself, therefore, offers the chance to relate to others in a respectful way in turn.

As John Rajchman argues, care of the self is thus implicitly ethical, yet not in a traditional sense of "finding the nature of the good life for Man and how to live it, or [of] determining the principle of our mutual obligations and how to follow it."[84] Care of the self is not an "ethic of prudence nor of duty."[85] Instead, care of the self is a commitment to exploring "who we are said to be" and experimenting with alternative possibilities.[86] It is an ethic that commits ourselves to ourselves ontologically, rather than either to a universalist deontological framework or to nihilistic relativities. Rajchman continues: "Foucault's philosophy was a philosophy neither of solidarity or objectivity. It was based neither in determining who we really are, nor in identifying with some one embattled group. Rather, in analysing the problematic ways we have been constituted as who we are, Foucault sought to raise questions about who we might become—in our thinking as in our lives."[87]

Losing Control of Social Media

In this book, we have explored how dominant views of living well on social media are equivalent to taking active control of your online habits for your own ends. Living poorly, on the other hand, is equivalent to letting platforms control your habits instead. We have seen how this constructs an ethics of active/passive use, whereby users are encouraged to get active on platforms, dominating technology to reach their own well-being goals, while not letting technology dominate their well-being through passive submission. In this way, social media is imagined as an empty vessel for the users' own intentions. If a user wants to engage with platforms responsibly—healthily—they can. Control is there for them to assume, if they want it. This binary, which maps onto wearisome structure-versus-agency debates, and corresponding tool-views of technology, renders a fairly stark ethical decision. Well-being on social media is framed to be a personal choice, and a personal choice alone, and the individual user is rendered solely responsible for their psychosocial experience of platforms, good or bad. This forecloses the opportunity to discuss how existing inequalities, marginalization, and other social determinants of health impact well-being online, or how the design of platforms themselves are also implicated in differentiated experiences of well-being. Through responsibilization, the user becomes entwined with moralized discourses of healthy and unhealthy behaviors, right and wrong forms of use. This book has revealed that it is through the articulation and enactment of these norms that the governance of well-being on social media is secured.

You might reasonably assume that taking back control of technologies like social media is a great example of how subjects can self-fashion themselves into something of their own choosing. A subject who wields technologies like social media for their own purposes. A subject who takes advantage of its possibilities to shape an indeterminate future of their own making. However, while appealing, such interpretations are built on shaky ground. Instead, the efficacy of care of the self on social media is better interpreted through alternative sociotechnical conceptualizations of technology, such as those that have underpinned the empirical analysis of this book. Rather than technology being something separate from the human—something that can, indeed, be controlled—the sociotechnical view considers technology as something much more fundamental, something much more entangled, and something much more co-constitutive of what it is to be a human being existing in the world at all.

Bruno Latour, for example, argues that "there is no sense in which humans may be said to exist as humans without entering into commerce" with the technical object that "authorises and enables them to exist (i.e. to act)."[88] By this, Latour is saying that technology facilitates human activity to such an extent that it is impossible to distinguish who or what is actually facilitating that activity to begin with—human or nonhuman, user or social media. In fact, for Latour, this distinction does not even make that much sense. Latour famously uses the example of the gun to advance this idea, which, to remind the reader, he calls *mediation*. You may be aware of the platitude, "Guns don't kill people, people kill people." In its logic, the gun is simply a tool that allows the person, as the primary agent, to kill another. The gun exists only as an object, through which the person's desire to kill flows. Here, much as with the tool-view of social media, humans are said to be in control of the technical object in order to enact their will. However, while simple, and while offering a comforting moral culpability, such a view is deeply misleading for Latour. Instead, Latour suggests that the gun effectively materializes a human desire to kill into the world by making it possible for that action to occur at that specific moment in time. The gun, therefore, translates a human desire for killing into action, without which the action simply would not have happened. This is transformative for Latour: "you are a different person with the gun in your hand," and the gun, by being in your hand, is different than if it were left snuggly in its rack.[89] Only when the human intention and the technical capacities of the gun are brought together can a shooting, as an observably discrete *human* action, actually take place.

Through this coming together of the human and the technical object, this *mediation*, it is impossible to neatly distinguish the primary agents of the scene. Crucially, this has implications for how we attribute morality to action. In this example, responsibility for the shooting—which can occur only through the combination of human and gun and, by proxy, those who produced and provided the gun—becomes shared. Who, then, is ethically and morally responsible here? Through the lens of mediation it is hard to say. Accountability for the issues that swirl around technology, as such, is also difficult to discern. While perhaps hard to put into practice in current liberal legal contexts, but not impossible, as recent work in *biolegality* suggests, these ideas of mediation force us to question common attributions of responsibility in our study of sociotechnical relations.[90] Returning to the topic of this book, and with this moral entanglement in mind, we may wonder how useful it is to think about social media in terms of either manipulation or control, of either unhealthy or healthy, of either bad or good. Maybe it is time to think of social media as less like an inanimate object, something that is either used for right or wrong. Instead, we could think of it as something much more profound and complex: as a generator of human morals, action, and will—as a fulcrum of well-being, even.

These questions surrounding mediation open an expansive problem space rather than giving simple answers. If nothing else, these ideas reveal that humans are, as they have been since they were born, in the thick of it, dependent on others and on objects to ensure the seemingly stable flow of their existence. You can't separate habits from technology, or technology from habits. Our activity on social media platforms—our likes, our shares, our comments—are thus not determined solely by design, yet they are not simply naturally occurring either. They are not automaton behaviors inculcated by nefarious companies, yet they are not strictly autonomous. And just as platforms do not exist without users, the user does not, and cannot, exist without platforms. As a result, neither individual users nor the manipulative design of platforms can be the sole causes of the well-being harms of social media, or the habits through which they are perpetuated. Rather, it is the coming together of human users and user interfaces, in specific localized settings, that coproduces any experiences of well-being that occur through them.

This coproduction has a significant impact for care of the self on social media. Specifically, properly considered practices of care of the self must reckon with the ways in which technologies shape, and are shaped by, the subject's thoughts and actions in various environments. For Jan Peter Bergen and Peter-Paul Verbeek, doing so is to take "socially situated technological artefacts seriously, recognizing the constitutive role they play in how we experience the world, how we act in it, and even the way we as subjects are constituted and can constitute ourselves."[91] For Verbeek, bringing these relations into focus through care of the self is a way to "stylize [our] moral subjectivity" with a clearer view.[92] In other words, to recognize the co-constitutive nature of technologies like social media is to better understand the various ways we are produced as subjects, and how we can produce ourselves in turn. Accordingly, for governed healthy users, and in the words of Lisa Nelson, this brings into focus the "methods, interests, materials, and institutions influencing" the design and dissemination of social media, while also acknowledging how users' own intentionality, modes of adaptation, and agentic action could alter their form in the future.[93]

For Steven Dorrestijn, the analysis of technical mediation thus "becomes a hermeneutic activity of exploring the influences on human existence," as they function as "part of the broader, ethical project" of determining varieties of conduct—both chosen and given.[94] For Dorrestijn, this indicates the existence of mediated, *hybrid* selves, fashioning and fashioned by the technological parameters of their lives. "Ethics," then, is not about "subjecting to technology, but about concern for the influences of technology and the wish to give style to our hybrid form of existence."[95] Care of the self, through the hermeneutic of mediation, can therefore help carve out an ethics of living well with social media beyond the restricting thresholds of autonomy, self-control, and responsibilization that characterize its present dominant form. In this way, care of the self on social media offers a way to move beyond the simplistic and reductive ideas of digital wellness we have encountered in this book, and the limiting political foreclosures and power relations such ideas perpetuate.

Again, and at the danger of repeating myself, the specific character of these new possibilities of social media well-being depends upon the situation, wishes, fears, demands, and hopes of each individual user. Nevertheless, in acknowledging the contingent, hybrid, mediated nature of their existence, users at least have the chance to change. Individuals may deem it fit to release themselves from some of the psychic burden that comes with the associated activities of being a healthy active user. They may also withhold judgment of others struggling to fulfill this role as well. Some may relax into their hybrid subject-position, taking comfort in the idea that their online activity is not entirely the result of their own will. They may seek to cultivate an easier relationship with social media as a result. Others may find the idea of being so enmeshed with social media's capitalist workings unbearable. They may extract themselves from online life altogether. Some may view their social media activity as only a small aspect of their well-being in general, dependent on much broader and pertinent forces of power, far beyond their own reach. Others may be galvanized by this insight and look to influence other levers beyond active use to attend to their future well-being, and the well-being of those in their community.

A Work of Fiction

Overall, the analytics and practices I have introduced above allow new forms of self-relation and action to emerge, producing changes in the form governance takes, revealing slight shifts in its points of pressure, and offering the chance for a new ethic of living well with social media to be formed. Offering care of the self as an alternative to dominant responsibilized views of social media well-being, and self-care in general, has been an attempt to ease some of the pressure felt by governed users to conform to its current parameters. Moreover, it has been my hope to encourage our intellectual attention toward imagining well-being in a more collective, politically engaged sense, one that takes into account how practices of mediation and relations of power are involved in its experience by differently situated users in the world today.

I have taken the stated obviousness of social media well-being as the point of departure for this book. We have examined where these ideas come from, how they are technically administered, and how they are personally felt. We have highlighted their functioning within forms of neuroliberal governance and platform capitalism. Through it all, we have shown how adopting active habits and practices of self-control is not simply equivalent to healthy use, but something that produces healthy users—users who fashion the ties that bind their own normalization. In doing so, and in an attempt to loosen these binds, we have proceeded with a specific objective in mind: "the problematization of the way we think about and judge certain objects in order to distance ourselves from their naturalness or self-evidence."[96] This has been intended to create new perspectives that could change "something in the minds of people," nothing more, nothing less.[97] Although a humble goal, and a goal some may think too vague for properly scholarly work, through it I have tried to respect the freedom of each reader (of each user, perhaps) to interpret my findings as they wish. Inescapably, as such, this potentiality leads to conceptual terrains I do not have the ability to conceive of myself. Moreover, it may produce ideas and practices about social media well-being far beyond what I would actually deem worthwhile.

In making room for this ambivalence, this book ought not be read in terms of either true or false, or really as an argument for one way of life over another. Instead, this book appeals to the different and direct experiences of each individual reader. Accordingly, we could better consider its impact in terms of fiction, most notably as an outcome "that one fabricates oneself" in relation to one's own life.[98] What this impact looks like, much as with well-being, will be different for different people. I hope to have offered a space for reflection that did not exist before for these different readers, opening something that will exist afterward, in different forms, and moving outward in indeterminate ways. Thus, for a book ostensibly about social media well-being, we can finally say that this book is not really about social media well-being at all. Rather, it is about exploring the various means through which we can create ourselves as thinking, living beings in the world, the current limits we encounter toward this end, and the ways we can move beyond them if we so wish.

Notes

Introduction

The epigraphs are from Meta Safety Center, "Mental Health & Well-Being—Digital Wellness," https://about.meta.com/actions/safety/topics/wellbeing/digitalwellness/ (accessed June 1, 2023), and Michel Foucault, *Archaeology of Knowledge* (New York: Routledge, 2002), 25.

1. John Dewey, *Human Nature and Conduct* (Henry Holt, 1922), 38.

2. Anthony L. Fisher, "Social Media Is a Parasite, It Bleeds You to Live," *Business Insider*, September 6, 2020, www.businessinsider.com/delete-social-media-phone-parasite-mental-health-instagram-twitter-facebook-2020-9; Lydia Keating, "I'm an Influencer, and I Think Social Media Is Toxic," *Slate*, February 1, 2022, https://slate.com/technology/2022/02/instagram-tiktok-influencer-social-media-dangers.html; Devi Sridhar, "Social Media Could Be as Harmful to Children as Smoking or Gambling—Why Is This Allowed?," *The Guardian*, July 4, 2023, www.theguardian.com/commentisfree/2023/jul/04/smoking-gambling-children-social-media-apps-snapchat-health-regulation.

3. Jason Cohen, "Tech Addiction Is Real: How to Cut Back on Screen Time and Wean Off Social Media," *PCMag UK*, May 12, 2023, https://uk.pcmag.com/ios/146827/tech-addiction-is-real-how-to-cut-back-on-screen-time-and-wean-off-social-media; Shira Ovide, "Are You Mindlessly Scrolling? Here's How to Tame Your Bad Tech Habit," *The Washington Post*, March 7, 2023, www.washingtonpost.com/technology/2023/03/07/taming-bad-tech-habbit/; The Chalkboard Editorial Team, "How Healthy Are Your Social Media Habits? 8 Tips To Upgrade Your Digital Wellness," *The Chalkboard* (blog), July 6, 2023, https://thechalkboardmag.com/healthy-social-media-habits/.

4. Emily B. O'Day and Richard G. Heimberg, "Social Media Use, Social Anxiety, and Loneliness: A Systematic Review," *Computers in Human Behavior Reports* 3 (2021): 100070.

5. Michel Foucault, "The Subject and Power," in Hubert L. Dreyfus and Paul Rabinow, *Michel Foucault: Beyond Structuralism and Hermeneutics* (Chicago: University of Chicago Press, 1983), 208–29.

6. Foucault, "Subject and Power," 221.

7. Bennett Cyphers and Gennie Gebhart, "Behind the One-Way Mirror: A Deep Dive into the Technology of Corporate Surveillance," Electronic Frontier Foundation, December 2, 2019, www.eff.org/wp/behind-the-one-way-mirror.

8. Jose van Dijck, "Datafication, Dataism and Dataveillance: Big Data between Scientific Paradigm and Ideology," *Surveillance & Society* 12, no. 2 (2014): 197–208.

9. Cristina Alaimo and Jannis Kallinikos, "Computing the Everyday: Social Media as Data Platforms," *The Information Society* 33, no. 4 (2017): 175–91.

10. Mark Whitehead, "Neuroliberalism in the Digital Age: The Emerging Geographies of the Behavioural State," in *Handbook on the Changing Geographies of the State*, ed. Sami Moisio et al. (Cheltenham, UK: Edward Elgar, 2020).

11. Mark Whitehead, Rhys Jones, Rachel Lilley, Rachel Howell, and Jessica Pykett, "Neuroliberalism: Cognition, Context, and the Geographical Bounding of Rationality," *Progress in Human Geography* 43, no. 4 (2019): 632–49, 633. This broad definition builds on Engin Isin's original introduction of the term, which focused more on the psychodynamics of neoliberal governance—especially the appeals to desire, emotions, and affect found in its aspirational discourses of individualism. Engin F. Isin, "The Neurotic Citizen," *Citizenship Studies* 8, no. 3 (2004): 217–35.

12. Philip Mirowski, *Never Let a Serious Crisis Go to Waste: How Neoliberalism Survived the Financial Meltdown* (London: Verso, 2014).

13. Studies of this are widespread and varied, yet Gershon's anthropological work is a great place to start: Ilana Gershon, "Un-Friend My Heart: Facebook, Promiscuity, and Heartbreak in a Neoliberal Age," *Anthropological Quarterly* 84, no. 4 (2011): 865–94; Ilana Gershon, "'Neoliberal Agency,'" *Current Anthropology* 52, no. 4 (2011): 537–55; Ilana Gershon, "Publish and Be Damned: New Media Publics and Neoliberal Risk," *Ethnography* 15, no. 1 (2014): 70–87.

14. Jim McGuigan, *Neoliberal Culture* (Basingstoke, UK: Palgrave Macmillan, 2016).

15. Wendy Brown, *Undoing the Demos* (Princeton, NJ: Zone Books), 2. Historically, neoliberalism has been linked to ordoliberal projects in post–World War II

Germany, the economic thought of Fredrich Hayek and Milton Friedman, and the fiscal practices of the International Monetary Fund and World Bank. These policy measures, along with a discursive focus on economic "growth" at all costs, have been prevalent in the Global North for the past four decades. See David Harvey, *A Brief History of Neoliberalism* (Oxford: Oxford University Press, 2005). For more on neoliberal logics (or reason), see Jamie Peck, *Constructions of Neoliberal Reason* (Oxford: Oxford University Press, 2010).

16. Peter Miller and Nikolas Rose, *Governing the Present: Administering Economic, Social and Personal Life* (Cambridge: Polity, 2008), 32.

17. Whitehead et al., "Neuroliberalism," 634.

18. Madeleine Akrich, "The De-scription of Technical Objects," in *Shaping Technology/Building Society: Studies in Sociotechnical Change*, ed. Wiebe E. Bijker and John Law (Cambridge, MA: MIT Press, 1992), 205–24.

19. For a good introduction to these widespread fields, see Aleena Chia, Ana Jorge, and Tero Karppi, eds., *Reckoning with Social Media* (Lanhan, MD: Rowman & Littlefield, 2021).

20. This is the idea that the designs of platforms and applications supplant user value with the interests of the shareholders of the company/product in question. See Colin M. Gray et al., "The Dark (Patterns) Side of UX Design," in *CHI '18: Proceedings of the 2018 CHI Conference on Human Factors in Computing Systems* (New York: Association for Computing Machinery, 2018), 1–14.

21. Pilkington describes neoliberalism as "not merely an intellectual edifice, but a continuous process of constructing a shifting reality, that of neoliberalization." Marc Pilkington, "Well-Being, Happiness and the Structural Crisis of Neoliberalism: An Interdisciplinary Analysis through the Lenses of Emotions," *Mind & Society* 15, no. 2 (2016): 226.

22. "Responsibilization involves the state encouraging or compelling individuals to acknowledge and assume a degree of responsibility for managing their own risks. This devolution of responsibility and the emphasis on self-management does not mean that the state has entirely lost interest in individuals' conduct. Responsibilization is not equivalent to anarchy nor is it entirely equivalent to self-help, although this might form a part of the process. Rather the neoliberal state legislates to establish the rules and boundaries for such self-management. In addition, the state seeks to increase the citizens' capacity for self-management because this is believed to best serve society's interests; responsibilization underscores the duty of the prudent and rational citizen to avoid becoming a burden on others." B. J. Brown and Sally Baker, *Responsible Citizens: Individuals, Health and Policy under Neoliberalism* (Cambridge: Anthem Press, 2012), 18.

23. Richard G. Wilkinson and Michael Marmot, "Social Determinants of Health: The Solid Facts," doc. no. EUR/ICP/CHVD 03 09 01, World Health Organization, Regional Office for Europe, 1998, https://apps.who.int/iris/handle/10665/108082.

24. Ben Golder, *Foucault and the Politics of Rights* (Stanford, CA: Stanford University Press, 2015), 35.

25. Golder, *Foucault and the Politics of Rights*, 35.

26. Michel Foucault, "Is It Really Important to Think? An Interview Translated by Thomas Keenan," *Philosophy & Social Criticism* 9, no. 1 (1982): 30–40, 35.

27. The original quote: "Things can be changed, fragile as they are." Foucault, "Is It Really Important to Think?," 35.

28. See Anna Alexandrova, "Well-Being as an Object of Science," *Philosophy of Science* 79, no. 5 (2012): 678–89; John Chambers Christopher, "Situating Psychological Well-Being: Exploring the Cultural Roots of Its Theory and Research," *Journal of Counseling & Development* 77, no. 2 (1999): 141–52; Guy Fletcher, *The Routledge Handbook of Philosophy of Well-Being* (New York: Routledge, 2015).

29. Conceptualizing well-being in different ways leads to different suggestions toward its improvement. For example, the eudaimonic approach, which focuses on the necessary ingredients of human flourishing, could focus on furnishing individuals with the requirements of the good life, whatever they may be. Hedonistic frameworks, which focus on the balance between pleasure and pain, may instead seek to encourage individuals to adopt the subjective behaviors that make them happy. Structural accounts, which aim to situate well-being within its material political context, may hope to change the environmental and social conditions within which an individual resides, perhaps through more concrete political means, in order to make life more equitable, and thus less stressful for them on a daily basis.

30. In an influential piece of work, Ng and colleagues write that "well-being is very much a collaborative project, which requires one to participate in a *cultural complex* and to attune oneself to the system of consensual understandings and shared practices in a certain cultural community." The authors argue that "what counts as well-being depends upon how the concepts of 'well' and 'being' are defined and practiced in different cultural communities." Aik Kwang Ng et al., "In Search of the Good Life: A Cultural Odyssey in the East and West," *Genetic, Social, and General Psychology Monographs* 129, no. 4 (2003): 317–63.

31. Sheila Jasanoff and Sang-Hyun Kim, eds., *Dreamscapes of Modernity: Sociotechnical Imaginaries and the Fabrication of Power* (Chicago: University of Chicago Press, 2015).

32. Jasanoff and Kim, *Dreamscapes of Modernity*, 4.

33. Nikolas S. Rose, *Inventing Our Selves: Psychology, Power, and Personhood*, revised ed. (Cambridge: Cambridge University Press, 2010).

34. Rose, *Inventing Our Selves*, 11.

35. Rose argues that the investigation of the human subject as a valid site of scientific measurement produces the human being as a particular "normal" type. Moreover, the categories through which this individual subject is measured necessarily relay the cultural norms of its historical milieu. In other words, the production of the psychological subject is always tied to a particular time and place and is therefore never a neutral scientific construction. See also the work of Danziger, who argues that the discipline of psychology "deals in test scores, rating scales, response distributions, serial lists, and innumerable other items" to select, expose, and compare individuals with others in a given field. Kurt Danziger, *Constructing the Subject: Historical Origins of Psychological Research* (Cambridge: Cambridge University Press, 2009), 2.

36. For some examples, see Seyedezahra Shadi Erfani and Babak Abedin, "Impacts of the Use of Social Network Sites on Users' Psychological Well-Being: A Systematic Review," *Journal of the Association for Information Science and Technology* 69, no. 7 (2018): 900–12; Ethan Kross et al., "Social Media and Well-Being: Pitfalls, Progress, and Next Steps," *Trends in Cognitive Sciences* 25, no. 1 (2021): 55–66; Philippe Verduyn et al., "Do Social Network Sites Enhance or Undermine Subjective Well-Being? A Critical Review," *Social Issues and Policy Review* 11, no. 1 (2017): 274–302; Patti M. Valkenburg, "Social Media Use and Well-Being: What We Know and What We Need to Know," *Current Opinion in Psychology* 45 (June 2022): 101294.

37. Patti M. Valkenburg, Irene I. van Driel, and Ine Beyens, "The Associations of Active and Passive Social Media Use with Well-Being: A Critical Scoping Review," *New Media & Society* 24, no. 2 (2022): 530–49.

38. Others suggest that active/passive use is too coarse a distinction, and misses the creativity, nuances, and variety of social media activity undertaken by different users for a variety of purposes. See Philippe Verduyn, Nino Gugushvili, and Ethan Kross, "Do Social Networking Sites Influence Well-Being? The Extended Active-Passive Model," *Current Directions in Psychological Science* 31, no. 1 (2022): 62–68.

39. Joanne V. Wood, "What Is Social Comparison and How Should We Study It?," *Personality and Social Psychology Bulletin* 22, no. 5 (1996): 520–37.

40. Adrian Meier and Benjamin K. Johnson, "Social Comparison and Envy on Social Media: A Critical Review," *Current Opinion in Psychology* 45 (June 2022):

101302; Laura Vandenbosch, Jasmine Fardouly, and Marika Tiggemann, "Social Media and Body Image: Recent Trends and Future Directions," *Current Opinion in Psychology* 45 (June 2022): 101289.

41. Sunkyung Yoon et al., "Is Social Network Site Usage Related to Depression? A Meta-analysis of Facebook–Depression Relations," *Journal of Affective Disorders* 248 (2019): 65–72.

42. Joseph B. Walther, "Social Media and Online Hate," *Current Opinion in Psychology* 45 (June 2022): 101298.

43. Soudeh Ghaffari, "Discourses of Celebrities on Instagram: Digital Femininity, Self-Representation and Hate Speech," *Critical Discourse Studies* 19, no. 2 (2022): 161–78.

44. Lara N. Wolfers and Sonja Utz, "Social Media Use, Stress, and Coping," *Current Opinion in Psychology* 45 (June 2022): 101305.

45. Leonard Reinecke et al., "Permanently Online and Permanently Connected: Development and Validation of the Online Vigilance Scale," *PLoS One* 13, no. 10 (2018): e0205384.

46. Lindsay M. Howard et al., "Is Use of Social Networking Sites Associated with Young Women's Body Dissatisfaction and Disordered Eating? A Look at Black-White Racial Differences," *Body Image* 23 (December 2017): 109–13; Anna Maaranen and Janne Tienari, "Social Media and Hyper-masculine Work Cultures," *Gender, Work & Organization* 27, no. 6 (November 2020): 1127–44.

47. Hae Yeon Lee et al., "Getting Fewer 'Likes' Than Others on Social Media Elicits Emotional Distress among Victimized Adolescents," *Child Development* 91, no. 6 (2020): 2141–59.

48. Mai-Ly N. Steers, Robert E. Wickham, and Linda K. Acitelli, "Seeing Everyone Else's Highlight Reels: How Facebook Usage Is Linked to Depressive Symptoms," *Journal of Social and Clinical Psychology* 33, no. 8 (2014): 701–31; Taina Bucher, "Want to Be on the Top? Algorithmic Power and the Threat of Invisibility on Facebook," *New Media & Society* 14, no. 7 (2012): 1164–80.

49. Fazida Karim et al., "Social Media Use and Its Connection to Mental Health: A Systematic Review," *Cureus*, June 15, 2020.

50. Betul Keles, Niall McCrae, and Annmarie Grealish, "A Systematic Review: The Influence of Social Media on Depression, Anxiety and Psychological Distress in Adolescents," *International Journal of Adolescence and Youth* 25, no. 1 (2020): 79–93; Adrian Meier and Leonard Reinecke, "Computer-Mediated Communication, Social Media, and Mental Health: A Conceptual and Empirical Meta-Review," *Communication Research* 48, no. 8 (2021): 1182–1209.

51. Relatedly, several scales of social media addiction have been devised to diagnose pathological modes of use that exacerbate these issues. For example, addiction is said to be an applicable diagnosis if social media engagement forms a dominating component of an individual's life, is used for mood modification, is compulsive, leads to withdrawal when discontinued, or creates interpersonal conflicts, among other factors. Maria Chiara D'Arienzo, Valentina Boursier, and Mark D. Griffiths, "Addiction to Social Media and Attachment Styles: A Systematic Literature Review," *International Journal of Mental Health and Addiction* 17, no. 4 (2019): 1094–1118.

52. Alberto Monge Roffarello et al., "Understanding Digital Wellbeing within Complex Technological Contexts," *International Journal of Human-Computer Studies* 175 (July 2023): 103034.

53. Linda K. Kaye, Amy Orben, David A. Ellis, Simon C. Hunter, and Stephen Houghton, "The Conceptual and Methodological Mayhem of 'Screen Time,'" *International Journal of Environmental Research and Public Health* 17, no. 10 (2020): 3661; Jonathan Haidt, *The Anxious Generation: How the Great Rewiring of Childhood Is Causing an Epidemic of Mental Illness* (London: Penguin, 2024).

54. Chantal Coles-Brennan, Anna Sulley, and Graeme Young, "Management of Digital Eye Strain," *Clinical and Experimental Optometry* 102, no. 1 (2019): 18–29; Xiaofei Guan et al., "Gender Difference in Mobile Phone Use and the Impact of Digital Device Exposure on Neck Posture," *Ergonomics* 59, no. 11 (2016): 1453–61. Here, difficulties sleeping are often linked to social media's tendency to exacerbate the fear of missing out (FoMO) or rumination over previous self-disclosures on platforms. Anushree Tandon et al., "Sleepless Due to Social Media? Investigating Problematic Sleep Due to Social Media and Social Media Sleep Hygiene," *Computers in Human Behavior* 113 (2020): 106487.

55. C.R. Blease, "Too Many 'Friends,' Too Few 'Likes'? Evolutionary Psychology and 'Facebook Depression,'" *Review of General Psychology* 19, no. 1 (March 2015): 1–13; Adrian Meier et al., "Instagram Inspiration: How Upward Comparison on Social Network Sites Can Contribute to Well-Being," *Journal of Communication* 70, no. 5 (2020): 721–43.

56. Cynthia A. Hoffner and Bradley J. Bond, "Parasocial Relationships, Social Media, & Well-Being," *Current Opinion in Psychology* 45 (June 2022): 101306.

57. Angela L. Falisi et al., "Social Media for Breast Cancer Survivors: A Literature Review," *Journal of Cancer Survivorship* 11, no. 6 (2017): 808–21.

58. Susan Abel, Tanya Machin, and Charlotte Brownlow, "Social Media, Rituals, and Long-Distance Family Relationship Maintenance: A Mixed-Methods Systematic Review," *New Media & Society* 23, no. 3 (2021): 632–54.

59. Mary Beth Oliver, "Social Media Use and Eudaimonic Well-Being," *Current Opinion in Psychology* 45 (June 2022): 101307.

60. Xiangyu Tao and Celia B. Fisher, "Exposure to Social Media Racial Discrimination and Mental Health among Adolescents of Color," *Journal of Youth and Adolescence* 51, no. 1 (2022): 30–44; Sakshi Ghai et al., "Social Media and Adolescent Well-Being in the Global South," *Current Opinion in Psychology* 46 (August 2022): 101318; Abigail Locke, Rebecca Lawthom, and Antonia Lyons, "Social Media Platforms as Complex and Contradictory Spaces for Feminisms: Visibility, Opportunity, Power, Resistance and Activism," *Feminism & Psychology* 28, no. 1 (2018): 3–10.

61. Moritz Büchi and Eszter Hargittai, "A Need for Considering Digital Inequality When Studying Social Media Use and Well-Being," *Social Media + Society* 8, no. 1 (2022).

62. Sandro Galea, Monica Uddin, and Karestan Koenen, "The Urban Environment and Mental Disorders," *Epigenetics* 6, no. 4 (2011): 400–4; Sungju Lim, Dumebi Nzegwu, and Michelle L. Wright, "The Impact of Psychosocial Stress from Life Trauma and Racial Discrimination on Epigenetic Aging—A Systematic Review," *Biological Research for Nursing* 24, no. 2 (2022): 202–15; Eric J. Nestler et al., "Epigenetic Basis of Mental Illness," *The Neuroscientist* 22, no. 5 (2016): 447–63.

63. My use of the term *Global North* in this book is an attempt to avoid making universalized claims about the experience of social media well-being across the world, and instead examine how habits are discussed and formed in relation to the demands of specific environments. Obviously, there are huge national, cultural, social, and economic disparities even within its remit, and its proposed purview is not unproblematic. Despite this, I am not seeking to reify the term, but rather employ it to draw attention to the specificity of my analysis, and acknowledge how this specificity functions within a geopolitical world order shaped by Eurocentric colonialism and the related epistemic violence wrought by academic anglophonic institutionalism. Moreover, this is not to say that the analysis of this book is irrelevant to the experience of those outside of these particular remits. Far from it, this book is meant to offer a point of comparison for any who are seeking some further clarity and different perspectives on its topics. See Afonso de Albuquerque, "The Institutional Basis of Anglophone Western Centrality," *Media, Culture & Society* 43, no. 1 (2021): 180–88; Fran M. Collyer, "Global Patterns in the Publishing of Academic Knowledge: Global North, Global South," *Current Sociology* 66, no. 1 (2018): 56–73.

64. Georgia Wells, Jeff Horwitz, and Deepa Seetharaman, "Facebook Knows Instagram Is Toxic for Teen Girls, Company Documents Show," *The Wall Street*

Journal, September 14, 2021, www.wsj.com/articles/facebook-knows-instagram-is-toxic-for-teen-girls-company-documents-show-11631620739.

65. Anna D. Gibson, Niall Docherty, and Tarleton Gillespie, "Health and Toxicity in Content Moderation: The Discursive Work of Justification," *Information, Communication & Society* 27, no. 7 (2024), 1441–57.

66. In these now common critiques, user attention is up for grabs on social media platforms, with many considering it to be in platforms' interests to keep the eyeballs of users on hosted content for as long as possible, in the hope that it drives up interactions. This builds on the idea that user attention is something that can be transformed into tangible data through activity, via processes of datafication, and then sold to interested third parties wishing to reach certain demographics of users with targeted messages across the web. For a useful critique on the concept, see Greg Elmer, "Prospecting Facebook: The Limits of the Economy of Attention," *Media, Culture & Society* 41, no. 3 (2019): 332–46. Terranova examines the concept in relation to the broader crisis of attentiveness in (consumerist) modernity, exploring the possibilities of *paying* attention as both a limiting and transformative practice. Tiziana Terranova, "Attention, Economy and the Brain," *Culture Machine* 13 (2012).

67. Joshua A. Braun and Jessica L. Eklund, "Fake News, Real Money: Ad Tech Platforms, Profit-Driven Hoaxes, and the Business of Journalism," *Digital Journalism* 7, no. 1 (2019): 1–21.

68. Markus Trengove et al., "A Digital Duty of Care: A Critical Review of the Online Safety Bill," SSRN, April 1, 2022, https://papers.ssrn.com/sol3/papers.cfm?abstract_id=4072593.

69. Paddy Leerssen, "Outside the Black Box: From Algorithmic Transparency to Platform Observability in the Digital Services Act," *Weizenbaum Journal of the Digital Society* 4, no. 2 (2024).

70. Gunn Enli and Karin Fast, "Political Solutions or User Responsibilization? How Politicians Understand Problems Connected to Digital Overload," *Convergence* 29, no. 3 (2023): 675–89.

71. In the context of the UK, where this is especially prevalent, Brown and Baker write: "Whilst the state has undertaken a withdrawal from many of the postwar consensus technologies for ensuring the health of its citizenry, this has been supplanted by a growth in discourse which places the responsibility for welfare squarely in the hands of citizens themselves. This has operated not so much through coercion but through exhorting citizens to undertake a variety of personal disciplines to manage themselves, arranging their bodies, minds and lives around the expert advice dispensed by public health bodies and government

agencies. Especially for those citizens deemed to be vulnerable or 'socially excluded,' notions of choice and responsibility are often accompanied by legislative frameworks through which their conduct can be regulated or normalized, and it is frequently supposed that a person's vulnerabilities arise as a result of poor personal decisions or bad habits." Brown and Baker, *Responsible Citizens*, 3–4.

72. Pat O'Malley, "Risk and Responsibility," in *Foucault and Political Reason: Liberalism, Neo-liberalism and Rationalities of Government*, ed. Andrew Barry, Thomas Osborne, and Nikolas Rose (Chicago: University of Chicago Press, 1996).

73. GOV.UK, "UK CMO Commentary on Screen Time and Social Media Map of Reviews," Department of Health and Social Care, February 7, 2019, www.gov.uk/government/publications/uk-cmo-commentary-on-screen-time-and-social-media-map-of-reviews.

74. "Healthy Social Media Habits," *NIH News in Health*, September 2022, https://newsinhealth.nih.gov/2022/09/healthy-social-media-habits.

75. Meta Safety Center, "Mental Health & Well-Being—Digital Wellness," https://about.meta.com/actions/safety/topics/wellbeing/digitalwellness/ (accessed June 1, 2023).

76. World Health Organization, "Social Determinants of Health," www.who.int/health-topics/social-determinants-of-health (accessed July 23, 2024).

77. Scholars from several disciplines have identified the way the social determinants of health intersect with class, gender, race, and level of education. See Michael Marmot and Richard Wilkinson, *Social Determinants of Health* (Oxford: Oxford University Press, 2005); Ruqaiijah Yearby, "Structural Racism and Health Disparities: Reconfiguring the Social Determinants of Health Framework to Include the Root Cause," *The Journal of Law, Medicine & Ethics* 48, no. 3 (2020): 518–26; Janki Shankar et al., "Education as a Social Determinant of Health: Issues Facing Indigenous and Visible Minority Students in Postsecondary Education in Western Canada," *International Journal of Environmental Research and Public Health* 10, no. 9 (2013): 3908–29. Others have questioned the social determinants of health framework, due to its breadth and potential vagueness. See M. Mofizul Islam, "Social Determinants of Health and Related Inequalities: Confusion and Implications," *Frontiers in Public Health* 7 (February 2019): article 11.

78. Marya and Patel, for example, extensively engage with this concept in their book *Inflamed: Deep Medicine and the Anatomy of Injustice*, while Rose, Birk, and Manning have examined the term in relation to *neuroecosociality*—which seeks to situate and examine differential experiences of mental health in relation to adverse environmental factors. See Rupa Marya and Raj Patel, *Inflamed: Deep*

Medicine and the Anatomy of Injustice (London: Allen Lane, 2021); Nikolas Rose, Rasmus Birk, and Nick Manning, "Towards Neuroecosociality: Mental Health in Adversity," *Theory, Culture & Society* 39, no. 3 (2022): 121–44.

79. Marya and Patel, *Inflamed*, 32

80. Marya and Patel, 29–70. Elsewhere, public health scholar Matt Fisher, for instance, writes: "Cumulative exposure to stressors over the life course correlates positively with worse physical and mental health outcomes, and differences in such exposure contributes to health inequalities between groups according to gender, race, and socioeconomic status." Matthew Fisher, "A Theory of Public Wellbeing," *BMC Public Health* 19, no. 1 (2019): 3.

81. Ann Cvetkovich, *Depression: A Public Feeling* (Durham, NC: Duke University Press, 2012); Sianne Ngai, *Ugly Feelings* (Cambridge, MA: Harvard University Press, 2007).

82. Tuomo Tiisala, "Foucault, Neoliberalism, and Equality," *Critical Inquiry* 48, no. 1 (2021): 23–44.

83. Tiisala, "Foucault, Neoliberalism, and Equality," 40.

84. Tiisala, 26–27.

85. Jeff Orlowski-Yang, dir., *The Social Dilemma* (film) (Boulder, CO: Exposure Labs, Argent Pictures, The Space Program, 2020); Center for Humane Technology, "Take Control of Your Social Media Use," August 17, 2021, www.humanetech.com/youth/take-control-of-your-social-media-use.

86. Nir Eyal, *Hooked: How to Build Habit-Forming Products* (London: Penguin, 2014).

87. Cherie Lacey, Alex Beattie, and Catherine Caudwell, "Wellness Capitalism and the Design of the Perfect User," *Interface Critique* 3 (2021): 127–50; Simone Natale and Emiliano Treré, "Vinyl Won't Save Us: Reframing Disconnection as Engagement," *Media, Culture & Society* 42, no. 4 (2020): 626–33.

88. Using Mark Fisher's cultural theory, Hoang and colleagues have critiqued such calls for digital detox as a "reflexively impotent (anti-)consumerism," responsive to apolitical inertia and politico-ideological hegemony. See Quynh Hoang, James Cronin, and Alexandros Skandalis, "Futureless Vicissitudes: Gestural Anti-consumption and the Reflexively Impotent (Anti-)consumer," *Marketing Theory* 23, no. 4 (2023). See also Ana Jorge, "Social Media, Interrupted: Users Recounting Temporary Disconnection on Instagram," *Social Media + Society* 5, no. 4 (2019); Trine Syvertsen and Gunn Enli, "Digital Detox: Media Resistance and the Promise of Authenticity," *Convergence* 26, no. 5-6 (2020): 1269–83.

89. The Center for Humane Technology, for example, acknowledges that placing the personal burden on individuals to change their habits alone is not

enough to ameliorate the problems that arise through the extractive social media ecosystem as a whole.

90. Richard H. Thaler and Cass R. Sunstein, *Nudge: Improving Decisions about Health, Wealth, and Happiness* (New Haven, CT: Yale University Press, 2008); Joram Feitsma and Mark Whitehead, "Behavioural Expertise: Drift, Thrift and Shift under COVID-19," *International Review of Public Policy* 4, no. 2 (2022): 149–70.

91. Rose, *Inventing Our Selves*, 10–11.

92. Rose, 10–11.

93. Roger Deacon, "Strategies of Governance Michel Foucault on Power," *Theoria: A Journal of Social and Political Theory*, no. 92 (1998): 113–48.

94. Daniele Lorenzini, "From Counter-conduct to Critical Attitude: Michel Foucault and the Art of Not Being Governed Quite So Much," *Foucault Studies*, no. 21 (June 2016): 7–21, 10.

95. As Nikolas Rose writes: "Governing in a liberal-democratic way means governing through the freedom and aspirations of subjects rather than in spite of them." Rose, *Inventing Our Selves*, 155.

96. Graham Burchell, "Liberal Government and Techniques of the Self," *Economy and Society* 22, no. 3 (1993): 267–82. For further works on the relationship and differences between governance and governmentality, see Graham Burchell et al., eds., *The Foucault Effect: Studies in Governmentality* (Chicago: University of Chicago Press, 1991); Mitchell M. Dean, *The Signature of Power: Sovereignty, Governmentality and Biopolitics* (London: SAGE, 2013); Michel Foucault, *Security, Territory, Population: Lectures at the Collège de France, 1977–78* (Basingstoke, UK: Palgrave Macmillan, 2007); Thomas Lemke, *Foucault, Governmentality, and Critique* (New York: Routledge, 2015).

97. Cadman writes: "This is why liberalism is the full art of governmentalisation, understood as an autonomous rationality (from sovereignty) and perpetual problematisation: must one govern? Do we govern too much? What is effective government?" Louisa Cadman, "How (Not) to Be Governed: Foucault, Critique, and the Political," *Environment and Planning D* 28, no. 3 (2010): 539–56, 548.

98. Sam Binkley, "Psychological Life as Enterprise: Social Practice and the Government of Neo-liberal Interiority," *History of the Human Sciences* 24, no. 3 (2011): 83–102; Michel Foucault, *The Birth of Biopolitics: Lectures at the Collège de France, 1978–79* (Basingstoke, UK: Palgrave Macmillan, 2010).

99. Michel Foucault, *On the Government of the Living: Lectures at the Collège de France, 1979–1980* (New York: Picador, 2016).

100. Foucault, "Subject and Power," 221.

101. This is as opposed to metaphorically cutting off the king's head in an act of final revolution.

102. Foucault, *Security, Territory, Population,* 18

103. Zizi Papacharissi, Thomas Streeter, and Tarleton Gillespie, "Culture Digitally: Habitus of the New," *Journal of Broadcasting & Electronic Media* 57, no. 4 (2013): 596–607.

104. This negative view of passive habit has generative comparisons with Kantian Enlightenment moral philosophy. For Kant, one of the main restrictive internal forces to rational human progress is habit. Habits are presented as threats to reason and, therefore, to cosmopolitan human *freedom.* Tony Bennett, "Habit: Time, Freedom, Governance," *Body & Society* 19, no. 2-3 (2013): 107–35. See also Charles Camic, "The Matter of Habit," *American Journal of Sociology* 91, no. 5 (1986): 1039–87; Clare Carlisle, "The Question of Habit in Theology and Philosophy: From Hexis to Plasticity," *Body & Society* 19, no. 2-3 (2013): 30–57.

105. Such a view limits the scope of the conversation about social media well-being to wearisome debates between technologically determinist thinking and its social constructivist rebuttal. Lisa Nelson has written a fantastic book that explores the limits and alternatives to these conceptualizations in regard to social media, largely drawing on post-phenomenological literature to do so. Lisa S. Nelson, *Social Media and Morality: Losing Our Self Control* (Cambridge: Cambridge University Press, 2018). For more on the post-phenomenological approach, see Peter-Paul Verbeek, *Moralizing Technology: Understanding and Designing the Morality of Things* (Chicago: University of Chicago Press, 2011).

106. Boaz Miller, "Is Technology Value-Neutral?," *Science, Technology, & Human Values* 46, no. 1 (2021): 53–80.

107. Michel Foucault, *The History of Sexuality, vol. 1: An Introduction* (London: Penguin, 1998), 82.

108. Foucault, *History of Sexuality, vol. 1,* 82.

109. Foucault encourages us to "move less toward a 'theory' of power than toward an 'analytics' of power: that is, toward a definition of the specific domain formed by relations of power, and toward a determination of the instruments that will make possible its analysis." Foucault, *History of Sexuality, vol. 1,* 82.

110. Michel Foucault, "The Truth and Power," in Michel Foucault and Colin Gordon, *Power/Knowledge: Selected Interviews and Other Writings, 1972–1977* (New York: Pantheon Books, 1980), 19.

111. Foucault, *History of Sexuality, vol. 1,* 92–93.

112. Giorgio Agamben identifies *apparatus* as a decisive technical term in the strategy of Foucault's thought. Agamben notes its appearance at the "intersection

of power relations and relations of knowledge," yet endeavors to bring our attention to the modes of subjectivation contained within it. The term *apparatus* "designates that in which, and through which, one realises a pure activity of governance devoid of any foundation in being." The apparatus, in this understanding, is a construct that seeks to fix the behavior of human beings along abstract formulations. Although all modes of human behavior can be said to be founded upon some sort of abstraction, the apparatus, for Agamben, is precisely a tool able to illuminate this groundlessness of being and, subsequently, offers a means for the individual to get to grips with the power relations that attempt to style the world as if this were not the case. In other words, the apparatus allows the individual to take note of the contingency of their historical situation despite the attempts of forces that would have it otherwise. Apparatuses, thus taken as abstractions, must necessarily work upon the human subject in such a way as to make it seem they fulfill a natural need. Agamben goes on to state that apparatuses "must always imply a process of subjectification, that is to say, they must produce their subject." The relationship between modes of knowledge, power, and subjectivation across a set of heterogeneous elements, the power relations and historical contingencies that *make* the human subject in time, therefore, is what is at stake when we employ the *apparatus* as a tool of critical inquiry. Giorgio Agamben, *"What Is an Apparatus?" And Other Essays*, trans. Stefan Pedatella and David Kishik (Stanford, CA: Stanford University Press, 2009), 3–11.

113. When asked in an interview in 1977 to define *apparatus*, Foucault answered: "What I'm trying to pick out with this term is, firstly, a thoroughly heterogeneous ensemble consisting of discourses, institutions, architectural forms, regulatory decisions, laws, administrative measures, scientific statements, philosophical, moral, and philanthropic propositions—in short, the said as much as the unsaid. Such are the elements of the apparatus. The apparatus itself is the system of relations which can be established between these elements. Secondly, what I am trying to identify in this apparatus is precisely the nature of the connection that can exist between these heterogeneous elements. . . . [T]here is a sort of interplay of shifts of position and modifications of function which can also vary very widely. Thirdly, I understand by the term 'apparatus' a sort of—shall we say—formation which has as its major function at a given historical moment that of responding to an *urgent need*. The apparatus thus has a dominant strategic function." Michel Foucault, "The Confession of the Flesh," in Michel Foucault and Colin Gordon, *Power/Knowledge: Selected Interviews and Other Writings, 1972–1977* (New York: Pantheon Books, 1980), 194–95.

114. Foucault, "Confession of the Flesh," 96.

115. Dean writes: "A *dispositif* is something like a network of relations between elements that responds to an emergency and that organises, enables, orients, fixes and blocks relations of force. It is simply an immanent ordering of a field of force according to a strategic function." Dean, *Signature of Power*, 50.

116. For Foucault, disciplinary power in particular is explicitly understood in tandem with habit. Habit, for Foucault, is the vehicle through which discipline takes root in sequestered individuals. Living in "a society of disciplinary power," as Foucault says, is to live in a society of apparatuses whose instrument is the "acquisition of disciplines or habits." Foucault argues that "instilling habits" within individual members of the population is a key instrument through which order and predictability are wrought in specific environments. Habit, for Foucault, is "what links one to an order of things, to an order of time and to a political order." The particular order Foucault is referring to in this instance is apparatuses of industrialized capitalist production. Foucault claims that our engagement with institutions of work, health, and education, among others, "produces a fabric of habits" through which the relations that hold the individual together with others in their shared milieu are fixed. Through "a play of coercion and punishment, apprenticeship and chastisement," Foucault says, the instilling of habits in individuals "produces something like the norm." This norm, bred and maintained through the disciplining of the subject through habits—habits that work upon both thought and action fused together in total experience, "is the instrument by which individuals are tied to the apparatuses of production." Michel Foucault, *The Punitive Society: Lectures at the Collège de France, 1972–1973*, ed. Arnold I. Davidson, trans. Graham Burchell (New York: Palgrave Macmillan, 2015), 237–39.

117. Carolyn Pedwell, "Habit and the Politics of Social Change: A Comparison of Nudge Theory and Pragmatist Philosophy," *Body & Society* 23, no. 4 (2017): 70.

118. Tony Bennett et al., *Assembling and Governing Habits* (Milton Park, UK: Taylor & Francis Group, 2021), 3.

119. Wendy Hui Kyong Chun, *Updating to Remain the Same: Habitual New Media* (Cambridge, MA: MIT Press, 2017), 8

120. Mariana Valverde, *Diseases of the Will: Alcohol and the Dilemmas of Freedom* (Cambridge: Cambridge University Press, 1998), 139.

121. Dewey, *Human Nature and Conduct*, 25–26.

122. Bruno Latour, "On Technical Mediation," *Common Knowledge* 3, no. 2 (1994): 29–64, 45.

123. Bruno Latour, "Where Are the Missing Masses? The Sociology of a Few Mundane Artifacts," *Shaping Technology/Building Society: Studies in Sociotechnical Change* 1 (1992): 225–58.

124. Bruno Latour, *Reassembling the Social: An Introduction to Actor-Network-Theory* (Oxford: Oxford University Press, 2005), 157.

125. Latour, "Where Are the Missing Masses?," 69.

126. Akrich, "De-scription of Technical Objects," 222.

127. Akrich, 222.

128. Akrich, 222.

129. Latour, "On Technical Mediation," 31–39.

130. This repurposing of concepts related to ANT perhaps requires further qualification. ANT is usually considered a descriptive rather than critical approach to the study of sociotechnical relations. Latour himself notably urged scholars to simply "just describe the state of affairs at hand" in sociotechnical networks, rather than engage in any assessments of the wider political, normative, or prejudicing effects of those networks for the human actors involved. In ANT, in fact, there are no *wider effects* beyond the network under analysis. However, organization scholars Whittle and Spicer argue that by remaining "indifferent about the specific means through which power is established" within and through actor-networks, such a claim of objectivity can actually be shown to reinforce "the state of affairs that it describes." According to Amsterdamska, moreover, the purely symmetrical focus of ANT, which treats human and nonhuman actors on an exactly equal footing, "eliminates all distinctions between the various means that can be used to achieve control over things or people." This aspect of ANT therefore makes it difficult, if not impossible, to talk of potentially unequal relations of power that flow through technical infrastructures, and inhibits critical judgments as to why such relations may be politically problematic. Therefore, for McLean and Hassard, "while ANT addresses the local, contingent and processual it fails to attend to broader social structures that influence the local"—all to the detriment of politically engaged critique. See Olga Amsterdamska, "Surely You Are Joking, Monsieur Latour!," *Science, Technology & Human Values* 15, no. 4 (1990): 495–504; Latour, *Reassembling the Social*; Chris McLean and John Hassard, "Symmetrical Absence/Symmetrical Absurdity: Critical Notes on the Production of Actor-Network Accounts," *Journal of Management Studies* 41, no. 3 (2004): 501; Andrea Whittle and André Spicer, "Is Actor Network Theory Critique?," *Organization Studies* 29, no. 4 (2008): 611–29, 626.

131. Matthew Fuller and Andrew Goffey, *Evil Media* (Cambridge, MA: MIT Press, 2012), 158.

132. Fuller and Goffey, *Evil Media*, 158–59.

133. Nelly Oudshoorn and Trevor Pinch, eds., *How Users Matter: The Co-construction of Users and Technology* (Cambridge, MA: MIT Press, 2003), 9; Steve Woolgar, "Configuring the User: The Case of Usability Trials," *The Sociological Review* 38, no. 1 (1990): 58–99.

134. Kjetil Fallan, "De-scribing Design: Appropriating Script Analysis to Design History," *Design Issues* 24, no. 4 (2008): 61–75.

135. This empirical attitude has resonances with André Brock's methodological approach of critical technocultural discourse analysis (CTDA), which, in brief, seeks to analyze technology as "discourse, practice, and artefact." Brock's work specifically centers underrepresented groups of technology users, such as African American Twitter users, to counter normative deficit perspectives that focus on "abnormal" use-cases or digital divides. In doing so, Brock emphasizes reading technology as text, a hermeneutic approach that "interrogates ideological influences within the technological artefact, within the practices incurred through the artefact's design, and within the discourses of that technology's users." André L. Brock, *Distributed Blackness: African American Cybercultures* (New York: New York University Press, 2020), 2–10.

136. Taina Bucher, *Facebook* (Cambridge: Polity, 2021).

137. Luke Stark, "Algorithmic Psychometrics and the Scalable Subject," *Social Studies of Science* 48, no. 2 (2018): 204–31.

138. Thaler and Sunstein, *Nudge*; Jessica Pykett et al., "Governing Mindfully: Shaping Policy Makers' Emotional Engagements with Behavior Change," in *Emotional States: Sites and Spaces of Affective Governance*, ed. Eleanor Jupp, Jessica Pykett, and Fiona Smith (London: Routledge, 2017), 69.

139. Whitehead, "Neuroliberalism in the Digital Age," 88.

140. Golder, *Foucault and the Politics of Rights*, 32.

141. Michel Foucault, "What Is Enlightenment?," in *Ethics: Subjectivity and Truth (The Essential Works of Foucault, 1954-1984, vol. 1)*, ed. Paul Rabinow (New York: The New Press, 1997), 319. At the beginning of "The Subject and Power," an essay written in 1982, Foucault attempts to thread together the overarching purpose of his work of the past decades: "I would like to say, first of all, what has been the goal of my work during the last twenty years. It has not been to analyse the phenomena of power, nor to elaborate the foundations of such an analysis. My objective, instead, has been to create a history of the different modes by which, in our culture, human beings are made subjects." Foucault, "Subject and Power," 208.

142. Stuart Hall, "Cultural Studies and Its Theoretical Legacies," in *Stuart Hall: Critical Dialogues in Cultural Studies*, ed. Kuan-Hsing Chen and David Morley (London: Routledge, 1996), 265.

Chapter 1

1. Gerry Greenstone, "The History of Bloodletting," *BC Medical Journal* 52, no. 1 (2010): 12–14.

2. Sherry Sayed Gadelrab, "Medical Healers in Ottoman Egypt, 1517–1805," *Medical History* 54, no. 3 (2010): 365–86.

3. Klaus Bergdolt, *Wellbeing: A Cultural History of Healthy Living* (Cambridge: Polity, 2008).

4. Greenstone, "History of Bloodletting."

5. Caragh Brosnan, "Epistemic Cultures in Complementary Medicine: Knowledge-Making in University Departments of Osteopathy and Chinese Medicine," *Health Sociology Review* 25, no. 2 (2016): 171–86.

6. Georges Canguilhem, *The Normal and the Pathological* (New York: Zone Books, 1991).

7. Canguilhem, *Normal and the Pathological*, 91.

8. Canguilhem, 77.

9. Canguilhem, 239.

10. Canguilhem, 239.

11. Nikolas Rose, *Politics of Life Itself: Biomedicine, Power, and Subjectivity in the Twenty-First Century* (Princeton, NJ: Princeton University Press, 2007).

12. Tuomo Tiisala, "Foucault, Neoliberalism, and Equality," *Critical Inquiry* 48, no. 1 (2021): 23–44.

13. Luke Stark, "Algorithmic Psychometrics and the Scalable Subject," *Social Studies of Science* 48, no. 2 (2018): 204–31.

14. Gerard Hanlon and Peter Fleming, "Updating the Critical Perspective on Corporate Social Responsibility," *Sociology Compass* 3, no. 6 (2009): 937–48.

15. Michel Foucault, "The Confession of the Flesh," in Michel Foucault and Colin Gordon, *Power/Knowledge: Selected Interviews and Other Writings, 1972–1977* (New York: Pantheon Books, 1980), 195.

16. Madeleine Akrich, "The De-scription of Technical Objects," in *Shaping Technology/Building Society: Studies in Sociotechnical Change*, ed. Wiebe E. Bijker and John Law (Cambridge, MA: MIT Press, 1992), 208.

17. Feminist scholars have demonstrated how the fixing of human roles in sociotechnical configurations often relays partial and gendered biases. For exam-

ple, Ellen Van Oost examined the demarcation of gender roles in electronic shavers, arguing that the design of the Philips Ladyshave and the Philishave, as sold in the United States from the mid-twentieth century, served to reinforce gendered constructs of the technologically averse, passive female user in contrast to the technically knowledgeable, active masculine user. This is evidenced, for Van Oost, in the masking of the technology of the Ladyshave, whereby the device was perfumed to cover the smell of oil, had no visible screws, and was marketed as part of a beauty set colored in pink, while the Philishave, conversely, had accentuated technical features, being designed to be self-serviceable, modifiable, and coming in a gunmetal and black colorway. Ellen Van Oost, "Materialized Gender: How Shavers Configure the Users' Feminity and Masculinity," in Nelly Oudshoorn and Trevor Pinch, eds., *How Users Matter: The Co-construction of Users and Technology* (Cambridge, MA: MIT Press), 193–208.

18. E. W. M. Rommes, "Gender Scripts and the Internet; the Design and Use of Amsderdam's [*sic*] Digital City," (PhD diss., University of Twente, 2002), 15.

19. Steve Woolgar, "Configuring the User: The Case of Usability Trials," *The Sociological Review* 38, no. 1 (1990): 58–99, 61.

20. Woolgar, "Configuring the User," 61.

21. Woolgar, 60.

22. Bryan Pfaffenberger, "Technological Dramas," *Science, Technology, & Human Values* 17, no. 3 (1992): 282–312, 291.

23. Helen Nissenbaum, "From Preemption to Circumvention: If Technology Regulates, Why Do We Need Regulation (and Vice Versa)," *Berkeley Technology Law Journal* 26, no. 3 (2011): 1367–86, 1377.

24. Special Counsel Robert Mueller had recently indicted the Russia-based Internet Research Agency on charges that Russian agents had appropriated individual profiles from US citizens and disseminated political disinformation and misinformation on Facebook. For details on the Cambridge Analytica case, see Carole Cadwalladr and Emma Graham-Harrison, "Revealed: 50 Million Facebook Profiles Harvested for Cambridge Analytica in Major Data Breach," *The Guardian*, March 17, 2018, www.theguardian.com/news/2018/mar/17/cambridge-analytica-facebook-influence-us-election.

25. Mark Zuckerberg, quoted from a video recording of the hearing found on *The Guardian Live* YouTube channel, "Mark Zuckerberg Testifies before Congress—Watch Live," streamed April 10, 2018, www.youtube.com/watch?v=mZaec_mlq9M.

26. Judith Butler, "Can One Lead a Good Life in a Bad Life? Adorno Prize Lecture," *Radical Philosophy*, no. 176 (2012): 9–18, 10.

27. Although Butler herself is perhaps critical of Foucault's notion of *subjectivation*, insofar as it denotes a "radical dependency" on the power relations through which the subject is made, the forms of self-relating that normative visions of the good life prompt have resonances with both thinkers' (anti-essentialist) accounts. Judith Butler, *The Psychic Life of Power: Theories in Subjection* (Stanford, CA: Stanford University Press, 1997), 83.

28. The metrification of affective interactions on social media, through affordances such as likes and emojis, works to "construct, stabilize, measure and evaluate any individual as an interpretable scalable subject." The results of these evaluations, Stark shows, provide ever more granular data for platforms to sell to interested third parties, increasing the data's value and sharpening the targeting of individualized messaging online, whether commercial, political, or otherwise. Stark, "Algorithmic Psychometrics and the Scalable Subject," 206.

29. Nikolas Rose, *Inventing Our Selves: Psychology, Power, and Personhood*, revised edition (Cambridge: Cambridge University Press, 2010), 11. Rose further writes that Western psychology emerged as a "coherent and individuated theoretical field" between the mid-nineteenth and early twentieth centuries. During this time, Rose argues that psychology tried to position itself as a "science of the human individual." Using the form of the psychological test corroborated alongside physiological examinations, psychological experimenters such as Gustave Fechner in Germany, Alfred Binet in France, and Francis Galton in Britain proposed a range of methods that could measure the distinct capacities of the individual human mind. Nikolas Rose, *The Psychological Complex: Psychology, Politics, and Society in England*, 1869–1939 (London: Routledge & Kegan Paul, 1985), 6.

30. Rose, *Inventing Our Selves*, 2.

31. Rose, 12.

32. Rose, 12.

33. *The Guardian Live*, "Mark Zuckerberg Testifies before Congress."

34. Nicholas Thompson, "How Facebook Checks Facts and Polices Hate Speech," *Wired*, July 6, 2018, www.wired.com/story/how-facebook-checks-facts-and-polices-hate-speech/.

35. Todd Spangler, "Facebook's Sheryl Sandberg: 'Not All Interactions in Social Media Are Equally Good for People,'" *Variety* (blog), February 28, 2018, https://variety.com/2018/digital/news/facebooks-sheryl-sandberg-social-media-well-being-1202713211/.

36. Meta for Developers, "Meta for Developers—From Consumption to Connection," https://developers.facebook.com/videos/f8-2018/from-consumption-to-connection/ (accessed August 24, 2023).

37. Meta, "Introducing Hard Questions," June 15, 2017, https://about.fb.com/news/2017/06/hard-questions/.

38. Meta, "Hard Questions: Is Spending Time on Social Media Bad for Us?," December 15, 2017, https://about.fb.com/news/2017/12/hard-questions-is-spending-time-on-social-media-bad-for-us/.

39. Ganaele Langlois and Greg Elmer, "The Research Politics of Social Media Platforms," *Culture Machine* 14 (2013).

40. Meta, "Hard Questions: Is Spending Time on Social Media Bad for Us?"

41. Moira Burke and Robert E. Kraut, "The Relationship between Facebook Use and Well-Being Depends on Communication Type and Tie Strength," *Journal of Computer-Mediated Communication* 21, no. 4 (2016): 265–81.

42. Susan Oman, *Understanding Well-Being Data: Improving Social and Cultural Policy, Practice and Research* (Cham, Switzerland: Palgrave Macmillan, 2021).

43. Burke and Kraut, "Relationship between Facebook Use and Well-Being Depends on Communication Type and Tie Strength," 66.

44. Roy F. Baumeister and Mark R. Leary, "The Need to Belong: Desire for Interpersonal Attachments as a Fundamental Human Motivation," *Psychological Bulletin* 117, no. 3 (1995): 497–529.

45. Bennett Cyphers and Gennie Gebhart, "Behind the One-Way Mirror: A Deep Dive into the Technology of Corporate Surveillance," Electronic Frontier Foundation, December 2, 2019, www.eff.org/wp/behind-the-one-way-mirror.

46. Forouzan Yazdanipoor, Hady Faramarzi, and Abdollah Bicharanlou, "Digital Labour and the Generation of Surplus Value on Instagram," *tripleC: Communication, Capitalism & Critique* 20, no. 2 (2022): 179–94.

47. Christian Fuchs, "Digital Prosumption Labour on Social Media in the Context of the Capitalist Regime of Time," *Time & Society* 23, no. 1 (2014): 97–123, 112.

48. Cristina Alaimo and Jannis Kallinikos, "Computing the Everyday: Social Media as Data Platforms," *The Information Society* 33, no. 4 (2017): 175–91.

49. Alaimo and Kallinikos, "Computing the Everyday."

50. Alaimo and Kallinikos, 187.

51. Alaimo and Kallinikos, 185–86.

52. Jason Raibley, "Health and Well-Being," *Philosophical Studies* 165 (2013): 469–89.

53. Philippa Foot, *Natural Goodness* (Oxford: Clarendon Press, 2001), 51.

54. Meta, "Bringing People Closer Together," January 12, 2018, https://about.fb.com/news/2018/01/news-feed-fyi-bringing-people-closer-together/.

55. Meta, "Bringing People Closer Together."

56. Michelle Murphy, *The Economization of Life* (Durham, NC: Duke University Press, 2017), 3.

57. Christian Fuchs, *Culture and Economy in the Age of Social Media* (New York: Routledge, 2015).

58. Bruno Latour, *Reassembling the Social: An Introduction to Actor-Network-Theory* (Oxford: Oxford University Press, 2005), 157.

59. Burke and Kraut, "Relationship between Facebook Use and Well-Being Depends on Communication Type and Tie Strength," 266.

60. Burke and Kraut, 67.

61. Sam G. B. Roberts and Robin I. M. Dunbar, "Communication in Social Networks: Effects of Kinship, Network Size, and Emotional Closeness," *Personal Relationships* 18, no. 3 (2011): 439–52.

62. Burke and Kraut, "Relationship between Facebook Use and Well-Being Depends on Communication Type and Tie Strength," 226.

63. Nicole B. Ellison et al., "Cultivating Social Resources on Social Network Sites: Facebook Relationship Maintenance Behaviors and Their Role in Social Capital Processes," *Journal of Computer-Mediated Communication* 19, no. 4 (2014): 855–70.

64. Pierre Bourdieu and Loïc J. D. Wacquant, *An Invitation to Reflexive Sociology* (Chicago: University of Chicago Press, 1992).

65. Meta, "Hard Questions: Is Spending Time on Social Media Bad for Us?"

66. Elise Klein et al., "Human Technologies, Affect and the Global Psy-Complex," *Economy and Society* 50, no. 3 (2021): 347–58.

67. Aníbal Quijano, "Coloniality of Power and Eurocentrism in Latin America," *International Sociology* 15, no. 2 (2000): 215–32.

68. Gayatri Chakravorty Spivak, *A Critique of Postcolonial Reason: Toward a History of the Vanishing Present* (Cambridge, MA: Harvard University Press, 1999).

69. Here, Facebook's attempt to situate its services within a neat lineage of human history can be considered a genealogy of sorts, one that demarcates appropriate inhabitation of the present by defining what the human *is*. This echoes Nietzsche's affirmation that the appropriation of the past by interested actors constitutes a direct intervention into present modes of being. Understandings of what we are, and where we come from, that is, implicitly establish where we ought to be going. Friedrich Nietzsche, *On the Genealogy of Morals: A Polemic*, trans. Michael A. Scarpitti (London: Penguin Books, 2013).

70. Michel Foucault, *Archaeology of Knowledge* (New York: Routledge, 2002), 73.

71. Phoebe Sengers et al., "Reflective Design," in *CC '05: Proceedings of the 4th Decennial Conference on Critical Computing: Between Sense and Sensibility* (New York: Association for Computing Machinery, 2005), 49–58.

72. Sengers et al., "Reflective Design," 49.

73. Hamid Ekbia and Bonnie Nardi, "The Political Economy of Computing: The Elephant in the HCI Room," *Interactions* 22, no. 6 (2015): 46–49.

74. Michel Foucault, *Discipline and Punish: The Birth of the Prison* (New York: Vintage Books, 1995).

75. Moira Burke, Robert Kraut, and Cameron Marlow, "Social Capital on Facebook: Differentiating Uses and Users," in *CHI '11: Proceedings of the SIGCHI Conference on Human Factors in Computing Systems* (New York: Association for Computing Machinery, 2011), 571–80.

76. Moira Burke, Cameron Marlow, and Thomas Lento, "Social Network Activity and Social Well-Being," in *CHI '10: Proceedings of the SIGCHI Conference on Human Factors in Computing Systems* (New York: Association for Computing Machinery, 2010), 1909.

77. Mark S. Granovetter, "The Strength of Weak Ties," *American Journal of Sociology* 78, no. 6 (1973): 1360–80.

78. D.W. Russell, "UCLA Loneliness Scale (Version 3): Reliability, Validity, and Factor Structure," *Journal of Personality Assessment* 66, no. 1 (1996): 20–40.

79. Burke, Marlow, and Lento, "Social Network Activity and Social Well-Being."

80. Michel Foucault, "The Subject and Power," in Hubert L. Dreyfus and Paul Rabinow, *Michel Foucault: Beyond Structuralism and Hermeneutics* (Chicago: University of Chicago Press, 1983), 208–29, 212.

81. William Davies, *The Limits of Neoliberalism: Authority, Sovereignty and the Logic of Competition* (London: SAGE, 2014).

82. Davies, *Limits of Neoliberalism*, 37 (emphasis in original).

83. Sam Binkley, "Psychological Life as Enterprise: Social Practice and the Government of Neo-liberal Interiority," *History of the Human Sciences* 24, no. 3 (2011): 83–102.

84. James S. Coleman, "Social Capital in the Creation of Human Capital," *American Journal of Sociology* 94 (1988): S95–120.

85. Gary Becker, *Human Capital* (New York: National Bureau of Economic Research, 1964); Theodore Schultz, "Investment in Human Capital," *American Economic Review* 51, no. 1 (1961): 1–17.

86. Coleman, "Social Capital in the Creation of Human Capital," 118.

87. Coleman, 97.

88. Emanuele Ferragina and Alessandro Arrigoni, "The Rise and Fall of Social Capital: Requiem for a Theory?," *Political Studies Review* 15, no. 3 (2017): 355–67, 358.

89. Michel Foucault, *The Birth of Biopolitics: Lectures at the Collège de France, 1978–79* (Basingstoke, UK: Palgrave Macmillan, 2010), 240.

90. Pierre Bourdieu, *Forms of Capital: General Sociology, vol. 3* (Cambridge: Polity Press, 2021).

91. Jo Littler, *Against Meritocracy: Culture, Power and Myths of Mobility* (London: Routledge, 2017).

92. Tiisala, "Foucault, Neoliberalism, and Equality."

93. B. J. Brown and Sally Baker, *Responsible Citizens: Individuals, Health and Policy under Neoliberalism* (Cambridge: Anthem Press, 2012), 18.

94. M. Mofizul Islam, "Social Determinants of Health and Related Inequalities: Confusion and Implications," *Frontiers in Public Health* 7 (February 2019): article 11.

95. Matthew Fisher, "A Theory of Public Wellbeing," *BMC Public Health* 19, no. 1 (2019): 3.

96. Sam Binkley, *Happiness as Enterprise: An Essay on Neoliberal Life* (Albany: State University of New York Press, 2014); Eeva Sointu, "The Rise of an Ideal: Tracing Changing Discourses of Wellbeing," *The Sociological Review* 53, no. 2 (2005): 255–74.

97. Ian Cummins, "The Impact of Austerity on Mental Health Service Provision: A UK Perspective," *International Journal of Environmental Research and Public Health* 15, no. 6 (2018): 1145.

98. NHS, "Live Well," January 17, 2022, www.nhs.uk/live-well/.

99. Wendy Brown, *Edgework: Critical Essays on Knowledge and Politics* (Princeton, NJ: Princeton University Press, 2005), 4.

100. Sarah Atkinson, "The Toxic Effects of Subjective Wellbeing and Potential Tonics," *Social Science & Medicine* 288 (November 2021): 113098.

101. Sarah Atkinson et al., "Being Well Together: Individual Subjective and Community Wellbeing," *Journal of Happiness Studies* 21, no. 5 (2020): 1903–21, 1909.

102. Atkinson et al., "Being Well Together," 1910.

103. Sarah C. White, "Relational Wellbeing: Re-centring the Politics of Happiness, Policy and the Self," *Policy & Politics* 45, no. 2 (2017): 121–36, 133.

104. White, "Relational Wellbeing," 133.

105. White, 133.

106. Atkinson et al., "Being Well Together," 1909.

107. Akrich, "De-scription of Technical Objects," 222.

108. Langlois and Elmer, "Research Politics of Social Media Platforms."

109. Tarleton Gillespie, "The Fact of Content Moderation; or, Let's Not Solve the Platforms' Problems for Them," *Media and Communication* 11, no. 2 (2023): 407.

110. Sara Ahmed, *The Promise of Happiness* (Durham, NC: Duke University Press, 2010), 167.

Chapter 2

The epigraphs are from Reuters, "Facebook Will Try to 'Nudge' Teens Away from Harmful Content," October 10, 2021, www.reuters.com/technology/facebook-will-try-nudge-teens-away-harmful-content-2021-10-10/; and Meta, "Health & Well-Being—Digital Wellness," https://about.meta.com/actions/safety/topics/wellbeing/digitalwellness/ (accessed June 1, 2023).

1. Richard H. Thaler and Cass R. Sunstein, *Nudge: Improving Decisions about Health, Wealth, and Happiness* (New Haven, CT: Yale University Press, 2008).

2. Thaler and Sunstein, *Nudge*, 4.

3. Meta, "Health & Well-Being—Youth Well-Being," https://about.meta.com/actions/safety/audiences/youth/health-well-being/ (accessed February 6, 2024).

4. Meta, "Health & Well-Being—Youth Well-Being."

5. Meta, "Health & Well-Being—Digital Wellness."

6. Ana Jorge, Inês Amaral, and Artur de Matos Alves, "'Time Well Spent': The Ideology of Temporal Disconnection as a Means for Digital Well-Being," *International Journal of Communication* 16 (2022): 22.

7. Niall Docherty, "Facebook's Ideal User: Healthy Habits, Social Capital, and the Politics of Well-Being Online," *Social Media + Society* 6, no. 2 (2020); Karin Fast, "The Disconnection Turn: Three Facets of Disconnective Work in Postdigital Capitalism," *Convergence* 27, no. 6 (2021): 1615–30; Anne Kaun, "Ways of Seeing Digital Disconnection: A Negative Sociology of Digital Culture," *Convergence* 27, no. 6 (2021): 1571–83.

8. Prior to his role at Meta, Nick Clegg was member of Parliament for Sheffield Hallam between 2005 and 2017. In 2010, after the UK general election resulted in a hung Parliament, the Liberal Democrat Party, led by Clegg, entered into a coalition with David Cameron's Conservatives to form a government. He then served as deputy prime minister beneath Cameron between 2010 and 2015. Infamously, one of the Liberal Democrat's preelection flagship manifesto policies

was a commitment to not increase undergraduate university student tuition fees. Yet in 2010, quickly after being elected, and in what many consider an "unprecedented . . . betrayal" of the first-time (mainly student) voters who voted for Clegg's Liberal Democrats, the coalition Parliament instead passed a motion to increase undergraduate fees in England from £3,290 to £9,000 per year, a rise of 174 percent. Peter Wilby, "By His Act of Betrayal, Clegg Will Lose His Greatest Reward," *The Guardian*, December 14, 2010, www.theguardian.com/commentisfree/2010/dec/14/betrayal-clegg-punish-alternative-vote.

9. Jonathan B. Wiener, "The Regulation of Technology, and the Technology of Regulation," *Technology and Science Entering the 21st Century* 26, no. 2 (2004): 483–500.

10. Subhabrata Bobby Banerjee, "Corporate Social Responsibility: The Good, the Bad and the Ugly," *Critical Sociology* 34, no. 1 (2008): 51–79; Sven Brodmerkel, "Should Brands 'Nudge Us for Good'? Towards a Critical Assessment of Neuroliberal Corporate Social Responsibility," *Journal of Public Affairs* 19, no. 1 (2019): e1898.

11. The utopian visions of technology and its potentially positive effects on human well-being is nothing new, as Dorrestijn and Verbeek show. Steven Dorrestijn and Peter-Paul Verbeek, "Technology, Wellbeing, and Freedom: The Legacy of Utopian Design," *International Journal of Design* 7, no. 3 (2013): 45–56.

12. Rafael A. Calvo and Dorian Peters, "Introduction to Positive Computing: Technology That Fosters Wellbeing," in *CHI EA '15: Proceedings of the 33rd Annual ACM Conference Extended Abstracts on Human Factors in Computing Systems* (New York: Association for Computing Machinery, 2015): 2499.

13. Jonathan M. Peake, Graham Kerr, and John P. Sullivan, "A Critical Review of Consumer Wearables, Mobile Applications, and Equipment for Providing Biofeedback, Monitoring Stress, and Sleep in Physically Active Populations," *Frontiers in Physiology* 9 (2018).

14. Dana Schultchen et al., "Stay Present with Your Phone: A Systematic Review and Standardized Rating of Mindfulness Apps in European App Stores," *International Journal of Behavioral Medicine* 28, no. 5 (2021): 552–60; Aatish Neupane et al., "A Review of Gamified Fitness Tracker Apps and Future Directions," in *CHI PLAY '20: Proceedings of the Annual Symposium on Computer-Human Interaction in Play* (New York: Association for Computing Machinery, 2020), 522–33.

15. Rebecca Jablonsky, "Meditation Apps and the Promise of Attention by Design," *Science, Technology, & Human Values* 47, no. 2 (2022): 314–36.

16. Ana Caraban et al., "23 Ways to Nudge: A Review of Technology-Mediated Nudging in Human-Computer Interaction," in *CHI '19: Proceedings of*

the 2019 CHI Conference on Human Factors in Computing Systems (New York: Association for Computing Machinery, 2019), 1–15.

17. Johan Redström, "Persuasive Design: Fringes and Foundations," in *Persuasive Technology*, ed. Wijnand A. IJsselsteijn et al. (Berlin: Springer, 2006), 114.

18. Redström, "Persuasive Design," 114.

19. This is a slightly different argument than the one posed by Langdon Winner in his piece "Do Artifacts Have Politics?" Winner inscribes technology with explicit functional aims that in some way determine their political interpretation; the vision of technology as part of a rhetorical dialogue remains more open. Nevertheless, the idea that technologies relay and reinforce the particular norms of their day, whether consciously endorsed by their designers or not, owes a great deal to Winner's thought. See Langdon Winner, "Do Artifacts Have Politics?," *Daedalus* 109, no. 1 (1980): 121–36.

20. B. J. Fogg, *Persuasive Technology: Using Computers to Change What We Think and Do* (Boston: Morgan Kaufmann, 2003).

21. Akrich, "The De-scription of Technical Objects," 208.

22. See, e.g., Cherie Lacey, Alex Beattie, and Catherine Caudwell, "Wellness Capitalism and the Design of the Perfect User," *Interface Critique* 3 (2021): 127–50; Laura Specker Sullivan and Peter Reiner, "Digital Wellness and Persuasive Technologies," *Philosophy & Technology* 34, no. 3 (2021): 413–24.

23. *The Guardian Live*, "Mark Zuckerberg Testifies before Congress—Watch Live," streamed on YouTube April 10, 2018, www.youtube.com/watch?v=mZaec_mlq9M.

24. Meta, "How Feed Works," Facebook Help Center, www.facebook.com/help/1155510281178725/?helpref=hc_fnav (accessed September 19, 2023).

25. danah boyd, "Facebook's Privacy Trainwreck: Exposure, Invasion, and Social Convergence," *Convergence* 14, no. 1 (2008): 13–20.

26. Alice E. Marwick and danah boyd, "I Tweet Honestly, I Tweet Passionately: Twitter Users, Context Collapse, and the Imagined Audience," *New Media & Society* 13, no. 1 (2011): 114–33.

27. Jayson Harsin, "Regimes of Posttruth, Postpolitics, and Attention Economies," *Communication, Culture and Critique* 8, no. 2 (2015): 327–33.

28. Ilana Gershon, "Un-Friend My Heart: Facebook, Promiscuity, and Heartbreak in a Neoliberal Age," *Anthropological Quarterly* 84, no. 4 (2011): 865–94

29. Michel Foucault, *Discipline and Punish: The Birth of the Prison* (New York: Vintage Books, 1995).

30. Taina Bucher, "Want to Be on the Top? Algorithmic Power and the Threat of Invisibility on Facebook," *New Media & Society* 14, no. 7 (2012): 1164–80.

31. Benjamin Grosser, "What Do Metrics Want? How Quantification Prescribes Social Interaction on Facebook," *Computational Culture*, no. 4 (November 9, 2014): S3.

32. Jessica Pykett et al., "Governing Mindfully: Shaping Policy Makers' Emotional Engagements with Behavior Change," in *Emotional States: Sites and Spaces of Affective Governance*, ed. Eleanor Jupp, Jessica Pykett, and Fiona Smith (London: Routledge, 2017), 69.

33. Mark Whitehead, Rhys Jones, Rachel Lilley, Rachel Howell, and Jessica Pykett, "Neuroliberalism: Cognition, Context, and the Geographical Bounding of Rationality," *Progress in Human Geography* 43, no. 4 (2019): 632–49, 633.

34. Mark Whitehead, "Neuroliberalism in the Digital Age: The Emerging Geographies of the Behavioural State," in *Handbook on the Changing Geographies of the State*, ed. Sami Moisio et al. (Cheltenham, UK: Edward Elgar, 2020), 188.

35. Will Leggett, "The Politics of Behaviour Change: Nudge, Neoliberalism and the State," *Policy & Politics* 42, no. 1 (2014): 3–19.

36. Daniel Pichert and Konstantinos V. Katsikopoulos, "Green Defaults: Information Presentation and Pro-environmental Behaviour," *Journal of Environmental Psychology* 28, no. 1 (2008): 63–73.

37. Hunt Allcott, "Social Norms and Energy Conservation," *Journal of Public Economics* 95, no. 9–10 (2011): 1082–95.

38. Herbert Alexander Simon, *Administrative Behavior: A Study of Decision-Making Processes in Administrative Organizations* (New York: Free Press, 1997).

39. Richard H. Thaler, *Misbehaving: The Making of Behavioral Economics* (New York: W. W. Norton, 2015).

40. Daniel Kahneman, *Thinking, Fast and Slow* (London: Penguin Books, 2012).

41. Riccardo Rebonato, "A Critical Assessment of Libertarian Paternalism," *Journal of Consumer Policy* 37, no. 3 (2014): 359.

42. Chad J. Valasek, "Disciplining the Akratic User: Constructing Digital (Un)Wellness," *Mobile Media & Communication* 10, no. 2 (2022): 235–50.

43. Thaler and Sunstein, *Nudge*, 6.

44. Thaler and Sunstein, 6.

45. Milton Friedman and Rose Friedman, *Free to Choose: A Personal Statement* (New York: Harcourt Brace Jovanovich, 1990).

46. Thaler and Sunstein, *Nudge*, 5.

47. David Halpern, *Inside the Nudge Unit: How Small Changes Can Make a Big Difference* (London: W. H. Allen, 2015).

48. Whitehead et al., "Neuroliberalism."

49. Whitehead et al., 633.

50. Anne-Lise Sibony, "The UK COVID-19 Response: A Behavioural Irony?," *European Journal of Risk Regulation* 11, no. 2 (2020): 350–57.

51. Wendy Brown, *Undoing the Demos* (Princeton, NJ: Zone Books), 21.

52. Brown, 20; Whitehead, "Neuroliberalism in the Digital Age," 188.

53. Whitehead, 188.

54. "Eat well, move more, live longer" was the slogan for the UK government's public health campaign to fight obesity, now subsumed within its "Healthier Families" campaign. "When the fun stops, stop" is a major campaign by the UK gambling industry to promote responsible betting, which remains prevalent despite its generally accepted lack of effectiveness. Philip W. S. Newall et al., "Impact of the 'When the Fun Stops, Stop' Gambling Message on Online Gambling Behaviour: A Randomised, Online Experimental Study," *The Lancet Public Health* 7, no. 5 (2022): e437–46.

55. Gerd Gigerenzer, "On the Supposed Evidence for Libertarian Paternalism," *Review of Philosophy and Psychology* 6, no. 3 (2015): 363.

56. Gigerenzer, "On the Supposed Evidence for Libertarian Paternalism," 375.

57. Gayatri Chakravorty Spivak, *A Critique of Postcolonial Reason: Toward a History of the Vanishing Present* (Cambridge, MA: Harvard University Press, 1999).

58. Gigerenzer, "On the Supposed Evidence for Libertarian Paternalism," 376.

59. Christoph Schneider, Markus Weinmann, and Jan vom Brocke, "Digital Nudging: Guiding Online User Choices through Interface Design," *Communications of the ACM* 61, no. 7 (2018): 67–73.

60. Schneider et al., "Digital Nudging," 68.

61. Schneider et al., 69.

62. Austin Carr, "How Square Register's UI Guilts You into Leaving Tips," *Fast Company*, December 12, 2013, www.fastcompany.com/3022182/how-square-registers-ui-guilts-you-into-leaving-tips.

63. Johan Egebark and Mathias Ekström, "Can Indifference Make the World Greener?," *Journal of Environmental Economics and Management* 76 (March 2016): 1–13.

64. James Turland et al., "Nudging towards Security: Developing an Application for Wireless Network Selection for Android Phones," in *British HCI '15: Proceedings of the 2015 British HCI Conference* (New York: Association for Computing Machinery, 2015), 193–201.

65. Min Kyung Lee, Sara Kiesler, and Jodi Forlizzi, "Mining Behavioral Economics to Design Persuasive Technology for Healthy Choices," in *CHI '11: Proceedings of the Sigchi Conference on Human Factors in Computing Systems* (New York: Association for Computing Machinery, 2011), 325–34.

66. Bruno Latour, "On Technical Mediation," *Common Knowledge* 3, no. 2 (1994): 29–64, 40.

67. Branden Hookway, *Interface* (Cambridge, MA: MIT Press, 2014), 1.

68. Hookway, *Interface*, 1.

69. Benjamin H. Bratton, *The Stack: On Software and Sovereignty*, Software Studies (Cambridge, MA: MIT Press, 2015); Hadler and Haupt, "Towards a Critique of Interfaces," in Florian Hadler and Joachim Haupt, eds., *Interface Critique* (Berlin: Kulturverlag Kadmos, 2016), 7.

70. Florian Cramer and Matthew Fuller, "Interface," in *Software Studies: A Lexicon*, ed. Matthew Fuller (Cambridge, MA: MIT Press, 2008), 151.

71. See works by Lev Manovich and Johanna Drucker for further studies on the interface and its generative effects. Johanna Drucker, *Graphesis: Visual Forms of Knowledge Production* (Cambridge, MA: Harvard University Press, 2014); Lev Manovich, *The Language of New Media* (Cambridge, MA: MIT Press, 2001).

72. Whitehead, "Neuroliberalism in the Digital Age," 188.

73. Meta, "Facebook Launches Additional Privacy Controls for News Feed and Mini-Feed," September 8, 2006, https://about.fb.com/news/2006/09/facebook-launches-additional-privacy-controls-for-news-feed-and-mini-feed/.

74. Matt Marshall, "Facebook Launches 'News Feed' and 'Mini Feed'—as YouTube Invades Turf," *VentureBeat* (blog), September 5, 2006, https://venturebeat.com/business/facebook-launches-news-feed-and-mini-feed-as-youtube-invades-turf/.

75. Meta, "Facebook Launches Additional Privacy Controls for News Feed and Mini-Feed."

76. Bucher, "Want to Be on the Top?"

77. Theresa Sauter, "'What's on Your Mind?' Writing on Facebook as a Tool for Self-Formation," *New Media & Society* 16, no. 5 (2014): 823–39.

78. Meta, "Bringing People Closer Together," January 12, 2018, https://about.fb.com/news/2018/01/news-feed-fyi-bringing-people-closer-together/.

79. Meta, "Bringing People Closer Together."

80. This is how Facebook describes its Ranking algorithm: "Your News Feed is made up of stories from your friends, Pages you've chosen to follow and groups you've joined. Ranking is the process we use to organize all of those stories so that you can see the most relevant content at the top, every time you open Facebook.

Ranking has four elements: the available inventory of stories; the signals, or data points that can inform ranking decisions; the predictions we make, including how likely we think you are to comment on a story, share with a friend, etc; and a relevancy score for each story." Meta, "Bringing People Closer Together."

81. Meta, "Bringing People Closer Together."

82. Meta, "Bringing People Closer Together."

83. The publication of this blog is dated after the HCI studies conducted by Facebook that were explored in chapter 1. This dating indicates that the decision to connect users to content they are most likely to interact with on the Feed can be linked to Facebook's research on healthy usership.

84. Meta, "Building a Better News Feed for You," June 29, 2016, *https://about .fb.com/news/*2016/06/building-a-better-news-feed-for-you/.

85. Meta, "Building a Better News Feed for You."

86. Meta, "Bringing People Closer Together."

87. Thereby relaying a similar eudaimonic conception of well-being I have identified in Facebook's construction of healthy, ideal usership so far.

88. Julian Morgans, "The Inventor of the 'Like' Button Wants You to Stop Worrying about Likes," *Vice* (blog), July 6, 2017, www.vice.com/en/article /mbag3a/the-inventor-of-the-like-button-wants-you-to-stop-worrying-about -likes.

89. Meta, "Like and React to Posts," Facebook Help Center, www.facebook. com/help/1624177224568554?helpref=hc_fnav (accessed September 19, 2023).

90. Carolin Gerlitz and Anne Helmond, "The Like Economy: Social Buttons and the Data-Intensive Web," *New Media & Society* 15, no. 8 (2013): 1348–65.

91. Meta, "Making News Feed an Easier Place to Connect and Navigate," August 15, 2017, https://about.fb.com/news/2017/08/making-news-feed-an-easier-place-to-connect-and-navigate/.

92. Meta, "Making News Feed an Easier Place to Connect and Navigate."

93. Jose van Dijck, "Datafication, Dataism and Dataveillance: Big Data between Scientific Paradigm and Ideology." *Surveillance & Society* 12, no. 2 (2014): 197–208.

94. Tarleton Gillespie, *Custodians of the Internet: Platforms, Content Moderation, and the Hidden Decisions That Shape Social Media* (New Haven, CT: Yale University Press, 2018); Ken Hillis, Susanna Paasonen, and Michael Petit, eds., *Networked Affect* (Cambridge, MA: MIT Press, 2015).

95. Michel Foucault, *The Punitive Society: Lectures at the Collège de France, 1972–1973*, ed. Arnold I. Davidson, trans. Graham Burchell (New York: Palgrave Macmillan, 2015), 237.

96. Alexander R. Galloway, *The Interface Effect* (Cambridge: Polity, 2012).

97. Hookway, *Interface*, 14.

Chapter 3

1. This interview study was granted ethical approval after being reviewed by the IRB Microsoft Research Ethics Review Program, which ensures all ethical considerations outlined by the Office for Human Research Protections.

2. Ben Light, Jean Burgess, and Stefanie Duguay, "The Walkthrough Method: An Approach to the Study of Apps," *New Media & Society* 20, no. 3 (2018): 881–900; Jean Burgess and Nancy K. Baym, "Twitter: A Biography," in *Twitter* (New York: New York University Press, 2020); Brady Robards and Siân Lincoln, "Uncovering Longitudinal Life Narratives: Scrolling Back on Facebook," *Qualitative Research* 17, no. 6 (2017): 715–30; Kristian Møller Jørgensen, "The Media Go-Along: Researching Mobilities with Media at Hand," *MedieKultur: Journal of Media and Communication Research* 32, no. 60 (2016).

3. Charles L. Briggs, *Learning How to Ask: A Sociolinguistic Appraisal of the Role of the Interview in Social Science Research* (Cambridge: Cambridge University Press, 1986), 2.

4. Mark Nichter, "Idioms of Distress: Alternatives in the Expression of Psychosocial Distress: A Case Study from South India," *Culture, Medicine and Psychiatry* 5, no. 4 (1981): 379–408; Mark Nichter, "Idioms of Distress Revisited," *Culture, Medicine, and Psychiatry* 34, no. 2 (2010): 401–16.

5. Nichter, "Idioms of Distress Revisited," 404. My gratitude to Dr. Rasmus Birk for first introducing me to the work of Nichter.

6. Bonnie N. Kaiser and Lesley Jo Weaver, "Culture-Bound Syndromes, Idioms of Distress, and Cultural Concepts of Distress: New Directions for an Old Concept in Psychological Anthropology," *Transcultural Psychiatry* 56, no. 4 (2019): 589–98.

7. Nikolas Rose, *Governing the Soul: Shaping of the Private Self*, 2nd ed. (London: Free Association Books, 1999).

8. Svend Brinkmann, "Languages of Suffering," *Theory & Psychology* 24, no. 5 (2014): 630–48.

9. Nichter, "Idioms of Distress," 379.

10. Kaiser and Weaver, "Culture-Bound Syndromes," 591.

11. Nichter, "Idioms of Distress Revisited," 404–8.

12. Norman Makoto Su, Amanda Lazar, and Lilly Irani, "Critical Affects: Tech Work Emotions amidst the Techlash," *Proceedings of the ACM on Human-Computer Interaction* 5, issue CSCW1 (April 2021): article 179.

13. Morten Axel Pedersen, Kristoffer Albris, and Nick Seaver, "The Political Economy of Attention," *Annual Review of Anthropology* 50, no. 1 (2021): 309–25, 310.

14. Yves Citton, *The Ecology of Attention*, trans. Barnaby Norman (Cambridge: Polity, 2017).

15. Raymond Williams, *Marxism and Literature* (Oxford: Oxford University Press, 1977), 232.

16. Alice Marwick, "The Public Domain: Surveillance in Everyday Life," *Surveillance & Society* 9, no. 4 (2012): 378–93.

17. Mai-Ly N. Steers, Robert E. Wickham, and Linda K. Acitelli, "Seeing Everyone Else's Highlight Reels: How Facebook Usage Is Linked to Depressive Symptoms," *Journal of Social and Clinical Psychology* 33, no. 8 (2014): 701–31.

18. Joe Deville, Michael Guggenheim, and Zuzana Hrdličková, *Practising Comparison: Logics, Relations, Collaborations* (Manchester, UK: Mattering Press, 2016), 33–38.

19. Sabina Pultz, "Shame and Passion: The Affective Governing of Young Unemployed People," *Theory & Psychology* 28, no. 3 (2018): 358–81.

20. Kate Henley Averett, "Queer Parents, Gendered Embodiment and the De-essentialisation of Motherhood," *Feminist Theory* 22, no. 2 (2021): 284–304.

21. Gina Neff and Dawn Nafus, *Self-Tracking* (Cambridge, MA: MIT Press, 2016); Jennifer B. Webb et al., "Downward Dog Becomes Fit Body, Inc.: A Content Analysis of 40 Years of Female Cover Images of *Yoga Journal*," *Body Image* 22 (September 2017): 129–35.

22. Bucher conducted interviews to see how Facebook users responded to the algorithmic ordering of their relationships on the platform, finding that engagement with Facebook's interface "generates a plethora of ordinary affects" in users. These affects included frustration, recalled by users who did not receive likes on their posts, surprise at being put into contact with forgotten friends, or happiness at being tagged in a photo by a member of their family. These various affective responses, for Bucher, demonstrate that the technological affordances of Facebook give users a "reason to react" on Facebook in a way that is productive of "different experiences, moods and sensations" in users. Bucher describes the production of novel user affects as becoming part of the "force-relations" of Facebook: generative moments weaving the emotional experience of users with particular technological functions. Taina Bucher, "The Algorithmic Imaginary: Exploring the Ordinary Affects of Facebook Algorithms," *Information, Communication & Society* 20, no. 1 (2017): 41–42.

23. Lee Humphreys, *The Qualified Self: Social Media and the Accounting of Everyday Life,* 1st edition (Cambridge, MA: MIT Press, 2018). Nicolette Little has further explored the negative implications of Facebook's Memories function in relation to the experience of survivors of gender-based violence. Nicolette Little, "Social Media 'Ghosts': How Facebook (Meta) Memories Complicates Healing for Survivors of Intimate Partner Violence," *Feminist Media Studies* 23, no. 8 (2023): 1–23.

24. Katrin Tiidenberg et al., "'I'm an Addict' and Other Sensemaking Devices: A Discourse Analysis of Self-Reflections on Lived Experience of Social Media," in *#SMSociety17: Proceedings of the 8th International Conference on Social Media & Society* (New York: Association for Computing Machinery, 2017).

25. Deborah Lupton, *Fat,* 2nd ed. (London: Routledge, 2018).

26. Julie Guthman, *Weighing In: Obesity, Food Justice, and the Limits of Capitalism* (Berkeley: University of California Press, 2011), 193.

27. Guthman, *Weighing In,* 193.

28. Nancy K. Baym, Kelly B. Wagman, and Christopher J. Persaud, "Mindfully Scrolling: Rethinking Facebook after Time Deactivated," *Social Media + Society* 6, no. 2 (2020).

29. Philippine Chachignon, Emmanuelle Le Barbenchon, and Lionel Dany, "Mindfulness Research and Applications in the Context of Neoliberalism: A Narrative and Critical Review," *Social and Personality Psychology Compass* 18, no. 2 (2024): e12936.

30. Jesper Aagaard, "Digital Akrasia: A Qualitative Study of Phubbing," *AI and Society* 35, no. 1 (2020): 237–44.

31. Michel Foucault, *The Birth of Biopolitics: Lectures at the Collège de France,* 1978–79 (Basingstoke, UK: Palgrave Macmillan, 2010).

32. Williams, *Marxism and Literature,* 11. Williams engages with Gramsci's notion of hegemony in his concept of structures of feeling. Refusing the totalizing abstractions of ideology as false consciousness, or worldviews as pure class domination, hegemony is distinguished by its state of flux, necessarily fabricated, managed, and maintained by certain groups. Subsequently, and crucially, the constructed contingencies of hegemonic relations are open to challenge through the proposal of alternative ordering relations by others. According to Gramsci, intellectuals have the potential to be at the vanguard of such counter-hegemonic practices by offering viable substitutes to the status quo—specifically through the development of what he calls *critical awareness.* This type of thought refuses to accept dominating frames of reference and instead seeks to create new ways of imagining the world and the individual and the role of community within it,

alongside the practical investigative techniques to do so. Antonio Gramsci, *The Modern Prince and Other Writings* (New York: International Publishers, 1959).

33. Zeena Feldman, "Quitting Digital Culture: Rethinking Agency in a Beyond-Choice Ontology," in Aleena Chia, Ana Jorge, and Tero Karppi, eds., *Reckoning with Social Media* (Lanhan, MD: Rowman & Littlefield, 2021), 103–27.

34. Feldman, "Quitting Digital Culture," 112.

35. Nick Seaver, "Captivating Algorithms: Recommender Systems as Traps," *Journal of Material Culture* 24, no. 4 (2019): 421–36.

36. Ulrich Dolata, "Privatization, Curation, Commodification," *Österreichische Zeitschrift für Soziologie* 44, no. 1 (2019): 181–97, 184.

37. Rahel Jaeggi, *Critique of Forms of Life* (Cambridge, MA: Belknap Press of Harvard University Press, 2018).

38. These feelings are often understood as "self-conscious emotions" in the psychological literature, along with others such as pride and humiliation. Guilt, shame, and embarrassment are conceptually very close, but, as we will see in the main text, distinctions can be made that offer fruitful and diverging paths of analysis. Jessica L. Tracy and Richard W. Robins, "Putting the Self into Self-Conscious Emotions: A Theoretical Model," *Psychological Inquiry* 15, no. 2 (2004): 103–25.

39. Tero Karppi, *Disconnect: Facebook's Affective Bonds* (Minneapolis: University of Minnesota Press, 2018).

40. Mariek M. P. Vanden Abeele, Annabell Halfmann, and Edmund W. J. Lee, "Drug, Demon, or Donut? Theorizing the Relationship between Social Media Use, Digital Well-Being and Digital Disconnection," *Current Opinion in Psychology* 45 (June 2022): 101295.

41. Leonard Reinecke and Adrian Meier, "Guilt and Media Use," in *The International Encyclopedia of Media Psychology*, ed. Jan van den Bulck and David R. Roskos-Ewoldsen (London: Wiley, 2020).

42. Peter N. Stearns, *Shame: A Brief History* (Champaign: University of Illinois Press, 2017).

43. Ana Jorge, "Social Media, Interrupted: Users Recounting Temporary Disconnection on Instagram," *Social Media + Society* 5, no. 4 (2019); Laura Portwood-Stacer, "Media Refusal and Conspicuous Non-consumption: The Performative and Political Dimensions of Facebook Abstention," *New Media & Society* 15, no. 7 (2013): 1041–57.

44. Judy Wajcman, *Pressed for Time: The Acceleration of Life in Digital Capitalism* (Chicago: University of Chicago Press, 2016).

45. Nancy Fraser and Rahel Jaeggi, *Capitalism: A Conversation in Critical Theory* (Cambridge: Polity, 2018), 19.

46. Fraser and Jaeggi, *Capitalism*, 19.

47. Fraser and Jaeggi, 19.

48. Andrew Milner, "Cultural Materialism, Culturalism and Post-culturalism: The Legacy of Raymond Williams," *Theory, Culture & Society* 11, no. 1 (1994): 43–73.

Conclusion

1. Michel Foucault, "What Is Enlightenment?," in *Ethics: Subjectivity and Truth (The Essential Works of Foucault, 1954–1984, vol. 1)*, ed. Paul Rabinow (New York: The New Press, 1997), 318.

2. Foucault, "What Is Enlightenment?," 318.

3. Foucault, 318.

4. Michel Foucault, "The Lives of Infamous Men," in *Power (The Essential Works of Foucault, 1954–1984, vol. 3)*, ed. James D. Faubion, trans. Robert Hurley (New York: The New Press, 2001), 172.

5. Foucault, "Lives of Infamous Men," 172.

6. Foucault, 172.

7. Michel Foucault, "The Subject and Power," in Hubert L. Dreyfus and Paul Rabinow, *Michel Foucault: Beyond Structuralism and Hermeneutics* (Chicago: University of Chicago Press, 1983), 208–29, 208.

8. Paul Rabinow, *Anthropos Today: Reflections on Modern Equipment* (Princeton, NJ: Princeton University Press, 2003), 19.

9. Foucault, "What Is Enlightenment?," 319.

10. Foucault, 319.

11. Kory P. Schaff, "Foucault and the Critical Tradition," *Human Studies* 25, no. 3 (2002): 323–32; Michel Foucault, *The Hermeneutics of the Subject: Lectures at the Collège de France 1981–1982* (New York: Picador, 2005), 12.

12. Foucault, "What Is Enlightenment?"

13. Foucault, "What Is Enlightenment?"

14. Immanuel Kant, "An Answer to the Question: What Is Enlightenment? (1784)," in *Practical Philosophy*, ed. Mary J. Gregor (Cambridge: Cambridge University Press, 1996), 11–22.

15. For D. W. Smith, "Foucault's philosophy recapitulated the three questions of Kant's philosophy: (1) What can I know? (What can I see and articulate within any given historical episteme?); (2) What can I do? (What power may I claim and what resistances may I counter?); and most importantly (3) What can I be? (How can I produce myself as a subject? How can I be otherwise? How can I think oth-

erwise?).” Daniel W. Smith, “Two Concepts of Resistance,” in *Between Deleuze and Foucault*, ed. Daniel W. Smith, Nicolae Morar, and Thomas Nail (Edinburgh: Edinburgh University Press, 2016), 268.

16. Amélie Rorty and James Schmidt, *Kant's Idea for a Universal History with a Cosmopolitan Aim: A Critical Guide* (Cambridge: Cambridge University Press, 2009).

17. Michel Foucault, “What Is Critique?,” in *The Politics of Truth*, ed. Sylvère Lotringer (Los Angeles: Semiotext(e), 2007), 32.

18. Thomas Lemke, “Critique and Experience in Foucault,” *Theory, Culture & Society* 28, no. 4 (2011): 26–48.

19. Michel Foucault, *The History of Sexuality, vol. 2: The Use of Pleasure* (New York: Vintage Books, 1990), 3–5. Beyond its phenomenological rendering, Foucault describes experience as “the correlation between fields of knowledge, types of normativity, and forms of subjectivity in a particular culture.” Again, notice the triangulation between knowledge, power, and ethics in play here.

20. Foucault, “What Is Enlightenment?,” 315.

21. Daniel Smith, “Foucault on Ethics and Subjectivity: ‘Care of the Self’ and ‘Aesthetics of Existence,’” *Foucault Studies*, no. 19 (June 2015): 135–50, 137.

22. Louisa Cadman, “How (Not) to Be Governed: Foucault, Critique, and the Political,” *Environment and Planning D* 28, no. 3 (2010): 547.

23. Judith Butler, “What Is Critique? An Essay on Foucault's Virtue,” in *The Political*, ed. David Ingram (Malden, MA: Blackwell, 2002), 226.

24. Jürgen Habermas and Seyla Ben-Habib, “Modernity versus Postmodernity,” *New German Critique*, no. 22 (1981): 3–14.

25. Charles Taylor, “Foucault on Freedom and Truth,” *Political Theory* 12, no. 2 (1984): 152–83.

26. Nancy Fraser, “Foucault on Modern Power: Empirical Insights and Normative Confusions,” *Praxis International* 1, no. 3 (1981): 272–87.

27. Butler, “What Is Critique?,” 226.

28. Michel Foucault, “Nietzsche, Genealogy, History,” in *Counter-memory, Practice: Selected Essays and Interviews*, ed. Donald F. Bouchard, 139–65 (Ithaca, NY: Cornell University Press, 2019).

29. Judith Butler, “Beside Oneself: On the Limits of Sexual Autonomy,” in *Undoing Gender* (New York: Routledge, 2004), 36–37.

30. Foucault, “Subject and Power,” 221.

31. Foucault, 221.

32. Foucault, “What Is Critique?,” 28 (emphasis in original).

33. Foucault elaborated the notion of the counter-conduct via his genealogy of Christian asceticism, tracing the broad movement from pastoralism to political governmentality in the West as a transition from the *economy of souls* to the *government of men*. Matthew Chrulew, "Pastoral Counter-conducts: Religious Resistance in Foucault's Genealogy of Christianity," *Critical Research on Religion* 2, no. 1 (2014): 55–65; Michel Foucault, *Security, Territory, Population: Lectures at the Collège de France, 1977–78* (Basingstoke, UK: Palgrave Macmillan, 2007).

34. Foucault, "Subject and Power," 221.

35. Foucault, 221.

36. Olga Demetriou, "Counter-conduct and the Everyday: Anthropological Engagements with Philosophy," *Global Society* 30, no. 2 (2016): 220.

37. Ben Golder, *Foucault and the Politics of Rights* (Stanford, CA: Stanford University Press, 2015), 154.

38. Arnold I. Davidson, "In Praise of Counter-conduct," *History of the Human Sciences* 24, no. 4 (2011): 25–41, 27.

39. Davidson, "In Praise of Counter-conduct," 27.

40. Foucault, "Subject and Power," 225.

41. Foucault, *History of Sexuality, vol. 2*, 30.

42. Smith, "Foucault on Ethics and Subjectivity," 41.

43. Smith, 41.

44. Raúl Fornet-Betancourt et al., "The Ethic of Care for the Self as a Practice of Freedom: An Interview with Michel Foucault on January 20, 1984," *Philosophy & Social Criticism* 12, no. 2–3 (1987): 112–31.

45. Diana Stypinska, *Social Media, Truth and the Care of the Self: On the Digital Technologies of the Subject* (Cham, Switzerland: Palgrave Macmillan, 2022), 7.

46. Recent work on care of the self and social media has sought to link these ancient practices to contemporary forms of platformed communication. Specifically, publishing content on social media has been examined in terms of *hupomnemata*, the ethopoietic writing of the self into existence. See Corinne Weisgerber and Shannan H. Butler, "Curating the Soul: Foucault's Concept of *Hupomnemata* and the Digital Technology of Self-Care," *Information, Communication & Society* 19, no. 10 (2016): 1340–55.

47. Fornet-Betancourt et al., "Ethic of Care for the Self as a Practice of Freedom," 122.

48. Fornet-Betancourt et al., 122.

49. Fornet-Betancourt et al., 122.

50. Michel Foucault and Graham Burchell, "Parrēsia," *Critical Inquiry* 41, no. 2 (2015): 219–53.

51. Foucault and Burchell, "Parrēsia," 245.

52. Stypinska, *Social Media, Truth and the Care of the Self*, 9.

53. Dana Richard Villa, *Socratic Citizenship* (Princeton, NJ: Princeton University Press, 2001), 58; Torben Bech Dyrberg, "Foucault on Parrhesia: The Autonomy of Politics and Democracy," *Political Theory* 44, no. 2 (2016), 271.

54. Peter Brown, *Power and Persuasion in Late Antiquity: Towards a Christian Empire* (Madison: University of Wisconsin Press, 1992).

55. Foucault and Burchell, "Parrēsia," 245.

56. Foucault and Burchell, 245.

57. Boris Traue, "The Cybernetic Self and Its Discontents: Care and Self-Care in the Information Society," in *Care or Control of the Self? Norbert Elias, Michel Foucault, and the Subject in the 21st Century*, ed. Andrea D. Bührmann and Stefanie Ernst (Cambridge: Cambridge Scholars, 2010), 158–78.

58. Fornet-Betancourt et al., "Ethic of Care for the Self as a Practice of Freedom," 118.

59. Besides the study of healthy social media users, the critical clarity offered through the related work of the limit attitude, the care of the self, and parrēsia has value for encounters with other ideal figures that percolate through everyday life, and that similarly offer normative points of reference for the individual to react to in their inhabitation. Consider ideals of the good student, the good girl, the good boy, the good citizen, the good wife, the good immigrant, the good worker, and so on. Although illustrative examples of a few arbitrary constructs, it is the shared interpretive ability to identify such ideal figures *as* ideal figures that is important here. Rendering such figures strange offers a chance to objectify whatever impact, negative or otherwise, they may be having in the various experiences of individuals in the world. This is not to level the huge disparities, respective risks, and threats of violence that failure to perform any of these different roles may carry in different locations. Equally, it is not to hypostatize their respective meaning or force for all individuals at all times. Rather, historicizing their construction through the limit attitude is a way to expose them as necessarily artificial edifices.

60. Michel Foucault, "Is It Really Important to Think? An Interview Translated by Thomas Keenan," *Philosophy & Social Criticism* 9, no. 1 (1982): 30–40, 35.

61. Holger Pötzsch, "Critical Digital Literacy: Technology in Education beyond Issues of User Competence and Labour-Market Qualifications," *tripleC: Communication, Capitalism & Critique* 17, no. 2 (2019): 221–40.

62. This fundamental question, for example, is something that concerned Adorno in the mid-twentieth century: the possibility of a good life in an inhumane world, one specifically wrought from the devastation of the Holocaust. See

Theodor Adorno, *Minima Moralia: Reflections on a Damaged Life*, trans. E. F. N. Jephcott (New York: Verso, 2005). Elsewhere, Marx's social critique of alienation is based on the abstraction of human *species-being* within capitalist labor relations. See Karl Marx and Frederick Engels, *Economic and Philosophic Manuscripts of 1844*, trans. Martin Milligan (Radford, VA: Wilder, 2011). More recently, the health implications of capitalism have been considered by public health scholars and psychologists. See, e.g., Rupa Marya and Raj Patel, *Inflamed: Deep Medicine and the Anatomy of Injustice* (London: Allen Lane, 2021); Bert Olivier, "Capitalism and Suffering," *Psychology in Society*, no. 48 (2015): 1–21.

63. John M. Roberts and Colin Cremin, "Prosumer Culture and the Question of Fetishism," *Journal of Consumer Culture* 19, no. 2 (2019): 213–30.

64. Byung-Chul Han, *Psychopolitics: Neoliberalism and New Technologies of Power*, trans. Erik Butler (New York: Verso, 2017).

65. Davidson, "In Praise of Counter-conduct," 32.

66. Davidson, 32.

67. Diana Stypinska, *On the Genealogy of Critique: Or How We Have Become Decadently Indignant* (Abingdon, UK: Routledge, 2020), 27.

68. Stypinska, *On the Genealogy of Critique*, 27.

69. Andrew Dilts, "From 'Entrepreneur of the Self' to 'Care of the Self': Neoliberal Governmentality and Foucault's Ethics," paper presented at the Western Political Science Association 2010 Annual Meeting,.

70. Trent H. Hamann, "Neoliberalism, Governmentality, and Ethics," *Foucault Studies*, no. 6 (February 2009): 37–59.

71. Fornet-Betancourt et al., "Ethic of Care for the Self as a Practice of Freedom."

72. Sara Ahmed, "Selfcare as Warfare," *Feministkilljoys* (blog), August 25, 2014, https://feministkilljoys.com/2014/08/25/selfcare-as-warfare/.

73. Lorde herself, as Ahmed recognizes, wrote about the tension between self-care and collective action, questioning whether the unwavering focus on the self inhibits the formation of the commonalities required for political struggle. Audre Lorde and Sonia Sanchez, *A Burst of Light: And Other Essays* (Garden City, NY: Ixia Press, 2017).

74. Ahmed, "Selfcare as Warfare."

75. For a good critical introduction to the dispersion of self-care throughout society, and how it builds on psychological forms of measurement, see William Davies, *The Happiness Industry: How the Government and Big Business Sold Us Well-Being* (London: Verso, 2015).

76. Jonathan Kaplan, "Self-Care as Self-Blame Redux: Stress as Personal and Political," *Kennedy Institute of Ethics Journal* 29, no. 2 (2019): 97–123.

77. Trisha Greenhalgh and Simon Wessely, "'Health for Me': A Sociocultural Analysis of Healthism in the Middle Classes," *British Medical Bulletin* 69 (2004): 197–213.

78. Maria Ishikawa, "Mindfulness in Western Contexts Perpetuates Oppressive Realities for Minority Cultures: The Consequences of Cultural Appropriation," *SFU Educational Review* 11, no. 1 (2018); Katie Gamby, Dominique Burns, and Kaitlyn Forristal, "Wellness Decolonized: The History of Wellness and Recommendations for the Counseling Field," *Journal of Mental Health Counseling* 43, no. 3 (2021): 228–45.

79. Talia Welsh, "The Affirmative Culture of Healthy Self-Care: A Feminist Critique of the Good Health Imperative," *IJFAB: International Journal of Feminist Approaches to Bioethics* 13, no. 1 (2020): 27–44.

80. Robert Paul Wolff, Barrington Moore, and Herbert Marcuse, *A Critique of Pure Tolerance* (Boston: Beacon Press,1969).

81. Fornet-Betancourt et al., "Ethic of Care for the Self as a Practice of Freedom," 118.

82. For a good introduction to this debate, see Hi'ilei Julia Kawehipuaaka-haopulani Hobart and Tamara Kneese, "Radical Care," *Social Text* 38, no. 1 (2020): 1–16; Susanna Rosenbaum and Ruti Talmor, "Self-Care," *Feminist Anthropology* 3, no. 2 (2022): 362–72.

83. Richard White, "Foucault on the Care of the Self as an Ethical Project and a Spiritual Goal," *Human Studies* 37, no. 4 (2014): 489–504.

84. John Rajchman, "Ethics after Foucault," *Social Text*, no. 13/14 (1986): 165–83, 166.

85. Rajchman, "Ethics after Foucault," 166.

86. Rajchman, 166.

87. Rajchman, 179.

88. Bruno Latour, "On Technical Mediation," *Common Knowledge* 3, no. 2 (1994): 29–64, 45.

89. Latour, "On Technical Mediation," 32.

90. Sonja van Wichelen and Marc de Leeuw, *Biolegality: A Critical Introduction* (Singapore: Springer Nature Singapore, 2024).

91. Jan Peter Bergen and Peter-Paul Verbeek, "To-Do Is to Be: Foucault, Levinas, and Technologically Mediated Subjectivation," *Philosophy & Technology* 34, no. 2 (2021): 325–48, 326.

92. Peter-Paul Verbeek, *Moralizing Technology: Understanding and Designing the Morality of Things* (Chicago: University of Chicago Press, 2011), 82.

93. Lisa S. Nelson, *Social Media and Morality: Losing Our Self Control* (Cambridge: Cambridge University Press, 2018), 7.

94. Steven Dorrestijn, "Technical Mediation and Subjectivation: Tracing and Extending Foucault's Philosophy of Technology," *Philosophy & Technology* 25, no. 2 (2012): 221–41, 236.

95. Dorrestijn, "Technical Mediation and Subjectivation," 236.

96. Michel Foucault, *Power (The Essential Works of Foucault, 1954–1984, vol. 3)*, ed. James D. Faubion, trans. Robert Hurley (New York: The New Press, 2001), 243.

97. Michel Foucault et al., eds., *Technologies of the Self: A Seminar with Michel Foucault* (Amherst: University of Massachusetts Press, 1988), 10.

98. Foucault, *Power*, 243.

Bibliography

Aagaard, Jesper. "Digital Akrasia: A Qualitative Study of Phubbing." *AI and Society* 35, no. 1 (2020): 237–44. https://doi.org/10.1007/s00146-019-00876-0.

Abel, Susan, Tanya Machin, and Charlotte Brownlow. "Social Media, Rituals, and Long-Distance Family Relationship Maintenance: A Mixed-Methods Systematic Review." *New Media & Society* 23, no. 3 (2021): 632–54. https://doi.org/10.1177/1461444820958717.

Adorno, Theodor. *Minima Moralia: Reflections on a Damaged Life*. Translated by E. F. N. Jephcott. New York: Verso Books, 2005.

Agamben, Giorgio. *"What Is an Apparatus?" And Other Essays*. Translated by Stefan Pedatella and David Kishik. Stanford, CA: Stanford University Press, 2009.

Ahmed, Sara. *The Promise of Happiness*. Durham, NC: Duke University Press, 2010.

———. "Selfcare as Warfare." *Feministkilljoys* (blog), August 25, 2014. https://feministkilljoys.com/2014/08/25/selfcare-as-warfare/.

Akrich, Madeleine. "The De-scription of Technical Objects." In *Shaping Technology/Building Society: Studies in Sociotechnical Change*, edited by Wiebe E. Bijker and John Law, 205–24. Cambridge, MA: MIT Press, 1992.

Alaimo, Cristina, and Jannis Kallinikos. "Computing the Everyday: Social Media as Data Platforms." *The Information Society* 33, no. 4 (2017): 175–91.

Albuquerque, Afonso de. "The Institutional Basis of Anglophone Western Centrality." *Media, Culture & Society* 43, no. 1 (2021): 180–88. https://doi.org/10.1177/0163443720957893.

Alexandrova, Anna. "Well-Being as an Object of Science." *Philosophy of Science* 79, no. 5 (2012): 678–89.

Allcott, Hunt. "Social Norms and Energy Conservation." *Journal of Public Economics* 95, no. 9–10 (2011): 1082–95. https://doi.org/10.1016/j.jpubeco .2011.03.003.

Amsterdamska, Olga. "Surely You Are Joking, Monsieur Latour!" *Science, Technology, & Human Values* 15, no. 4 (1990): 495–504.

Atkinson, Sarah. "The Toxic Effects of Subjective Wellbeing and Potential Tonics." *Social Science & Medicine* 288 (November 2021): 113098. https:// doi.org/10.1016/j.socscimed.2020.113098.

Atkinson, Sarah, Anne-Marie Bagnall, Rhiannon Corcoran, Jane South, and Sarah Curtis. "Being Well Together: Individual Subjective and Community Wellbeing." *Journal of Happiness Studies* 21, no. 5 (2020): 1903–21. https:// doi.org/10.1007/s10902-019-00146-2.

Averett, Kate Henley. "Queer Parents, Gendered Embodiment and the De-essentialisation of Motherhood." *Feminist Theory* 22, no. 2 (2021): 284–304. https://doi.org/10.1177/1464700121989226.

Banerjee, Subhabrata Bobby. "Corporate Social Responsibility: The Good, the Bad and the Ugly." *Critical Sociology* 34, no. 1 (2008): 51–79. https://doi.org /10.1177/0896920507084623.

Barry, Andrew, Thomas Osborne, and Nikolas Rose, eds. *Foucault and Political Reason: Liberalism, Neo-Liberalism and the Rationalities of Government.* Chicago: University of Chicago Press, 1996.

Baumeister, Roy F., and Mark R. Leary. "The Need to Belong: Desire for Interpersonal Attachments as a Fundamental Human Motivation." *Psychological Bulletin* 117, no. 3 (1995): 497–529. https://doi.org/10.1037/0033-2909.117.3.497.

Baym, Nancy K., Kelly B. Wagman, and Christopher J. Persaud. "Mindfully Scrolling: Rethinking Facebook after Time Deactivated." *Social Media + Society* 6, no. 2 (2020): 2056305120919105. https://doi.org/10.1177 /2056305120919105.

Becker, G. *Human Capital.* New York: National Bureau of Economic Research, 1964.

Bennett, Tony. "Habit: Time, Freedom, Governance." *Body & Society* 19, no. 2–3 (2013): 107–35. https://doi.org/10.1177/1357034X13475828.

Bennett, Tony, Ben Dibley, Gay Hawkins, and Greg Noble. *Assembling and Governing Habits.* Milton Park, UK: Taylor & Francis Group, 2021.

Bergdolt, Klaus. *Wellbeing: A Cultural History of Healthy Living.* Cambridge: Polity, 2008.

Bergen, Jan Peter, and Peter-Paul Verbeek. "To-Do Is to Be: Foucault, Levinas, and Technologically Mediated Subjectivation." *Philosophy & Technology* 34, no. 2 (2021): 325–48. https://doi.org/10.1007/s13347-019-00390-7.

Binkley, Sam. *Happiness as Enterprise: An Essay on Neoliberal Life*. Albany: State University of New York Press, 2014.

———. "Psychological Life as Enterprise: Social Practice and the Government of Neo-liberal Interiority." *History of the Human Sciences* 24, no. 3 (2011): 83–102. https://doi.org/10.1177/0952695111412877.

Blease, C. R. "Too Many 'Friends,' Too Few 'Likes'? Evolutionary Psychology and 'Facebook Depression.'" *Review of General Psychology* 19, no. 1 (2015): 1–13. https://doi.org/10.1037/gpr0000030.

Bourdieu, Pierre. *Forms of Capital: General Sociology, vol. 3*. Cambridge: Polity, 2021.

Bourdieu, Pierre, and Loïc J. D. Wacquant. *An Invitation to Reflexive Sociology*. Chicago: University of Chicago Press, 1992.

boyd, danah. "Facebook's Privacy Trainwreck: Exposure, Invasion, and Social Convergence." *Convergence* 14, no. 1 (2008): 13–20. https://doi.org/10.1177/1354856507084416.

Bratton, Benjamin H. *The Stack: On Software and Sovereignty*. Software Studies. Cambridge, MA: MIT Press, 2015.

Braun, Joshua A., and Jessica L. Eklund. "Fake News, Real Money: Ad Tech Platforms, Profit-Driven Hoaxes, and the Business of Journalism." *Digital Journalism* 7, no. 1 (2019): 1–21. https://doi.org/10.1080/21670811.2018.1556314.

Briggs, Charles L. *Learning How to Ask: A Sociolinguistic Appraisal of the Role of the Interview in Social Science Research*. Cambridge: Cambridge University Press, 1986.

Brinkmann, Svend. "Languages of Suffering." *Theory & Psychology* 24, no. 5 (2014): 630–48. https://doi.org/10.1177/0959354314531523.

Brock, André L. *Distributed Blackness: African American Cybercultures*. New York: New York University Press, 2020.

Brodmerkel, Sven. "Should Brands 'Nudge Us for Good'? Towards a Critical Assessment of Neuro-liberal Corporate Social Responsibility." *Journal of Public Affairs* 19, no. 1 (2019): e1898. https://doi.org/10.1002/pa.1898.

Brosnan, Caragh. "Epistemic Cultures in Complementary Medicine: Knowledge-Making in University Departments of Osteopathy and Chinese Medicine." *Health Sociology Review* 25, no. 2 (2016): 171–86. https://doi.org/10.1080/14461242.2016.1171161.

Brown, B. J., and Sally Baker. *Responsible Citizens: Individuals, Health and Policy under Neoliberalism*. Cambridge: Anthem Press, 2012.

Brown, Peter. *Power and Persuasion in Late Antiquity: Towards a Christian Empire*. Madison: University of Wisconsin Press, 1992.

Brown, Wendy. *Edgework: Critical Essays on Knowledge and Politics*. Princeton, NJ: Princeton University Press, 2005.

———. *Undoing the Demos: Neoliberalism's Stealth Revolution*. Princeton, NJ: Zone Books, 2015.

Bucher, Taina. "The Algorithmic Imaginary: Exploring the Ordinary Affects of Facebook Algorithms." *Information, Communication & Society* 20, no. 1 (2017): 30–44. https://doi.org/10.1080/1369118X.2016.1154086.

———. *Facebook*. Cambridge: Polity, 2021.

———. "Want to Be on the Top? Algorithmic Power and the Threat of Invisibility on Facebook." *New Media & Society* 14, no. 7 (2012): 1164–80. https://doi .org/10.1177/1461444812440159.

Büchi, Moritz, and Eszter Hargittai. "A Need for Considering Digital Inequality When Studying Social Media Use and Well-Being." *Social Media + Society* 8, no. 1 (2022): https://doi.org/10.1177/20563051211069125.

Burchell, Graham. "Liberal Government and Techniques of the Self." *Economy and Society* 22, no. 3 (1993): 267–82. https://doi.org/10.1080 /03085149300000018.

Burchell, Graham, Colin Gordon, and Peter Miller, eds. *The Foucault Effect: Studies in Governmentality*. Chicago: University of Chicago Press, 1991.

Burgess, Jean, and Nancy K. Baym. "Twitter: A Biography." In *Twitter*. New York: New York University Press, 2020.

Burke, Moira, and Robert E. Kraut. "The Relationship between Facebook Use and Well-Being Depends on Communication Type and Tie Strength." *Journal of Computer-Mediated Communication* 21, no. 4 (2016): 265–81. https://doi.org/10.1111/jcc4.12162.

Burke, Moira, Robert Kraut, and Cameron Marlow. "Social Capital on Facebook: Differentiating Uses and Users." In *CHI '11: Proceedings of the SIGCHI Conference on Human Factors in Computing Systems*, 571–80. New York: Association for Computing Machinery, 2011. https://doi.org/10.1145 /1978942.1979023.

Burke, Moira, Cameron Marlow, and Thomas Lento. "Social Network Activity and Social Well-Being." In *CHI '10: Proceedings of the SIGCHI Conference on Human Factors in Computing Systems*, 1909–12. New York: Association for Computing Machinery, 2010. https://doi.org/10.1145/1753326.1753613.

Butler, Judith. "Can One Lead a Good Life in a Bad Life? Adorno Prize Lecture." *Radical Philosophy*, no. 176 (2012): 9–18.

———. *The Psychic Life of Power: Theories in Subjection.* Stanford, CA: Stanford University Press, 1997.

———. *Undoing Gender.* London: Routledge, 2004.

———. "What Is Critique? An Essay on Foucault's Virtue." In *The Political*, edited by David Ingram. Malden, MA: Blackwell, 2002.

Cadman, Louisa. "How (Not) to Be Governed: Foucault, Critique, and the Political." *Environment and Planning D* 28, no. 3 (2010): 539–56. https://doi.org/10.1068/d4509.

Cadwalladr, Carole, and Emma Graham-Harrison. "Revealed: 50 Million Facebook Profiles Harvested for Cambridge Analytica in Major Data Breach." *The Guardian*, March 17, 2018. www.theguardian.com/news/2018/mar/17/cambridge-analytica-facebook-influence-us-election.

Calvo, Rafael A., and Dorian Peters. "Introduction to Positive Computing: Technology That Fosters Wellbeing." In *Proceedings of the 33rd Annual ACM Conference Extended Abstracts on Human Factors in Computing Systems*, 2499–2500. CHI EA '15. New York: Association for Computing Machinery, 2015. https://doi.org/10.1145/2702613.2706674.

Camic, Charles. "The Matter of Habit." *American Journal of Sociology* 91, no. 5 (1986): 1039–87.

Canguilhem, Georges. *The Normal and the Pathological.* New York: Zone Books, 1991.

Caraban, Ana, Evangelos Karapanos, Daniel Gonçalves, and Pedro Campos. "23 Ways to Nudge: A Review of Technology-Mediated Nudging in Human-Computer Interaction." In *CHI '19: Proceedings of the 2019 CHI Conference on Human Factors in Computing Systems*, 1–15. New York: Association for Computing Machinery, 2019. https://doi.org/10.1145/3290605.3300733.

Carlisle, Clare. "The Question of Habit in Theology and Philosophy: From Hexis to Plasticity." *Body & Society* 19, no. 2–3 (2013): 30–57. https://doi.org/10.1177/1357034X12474475.

Carr, Austin. "How Square Register's UI Guilts You into Leaving Tips." *Fast Company*, December 12, 2013. www.fastcompany.com/3022182/how-square-registers-ui-guilts-you-into-leaving-tips.

Chachignon, Philippine, Emmanuelle Le Barbenchon, and Lionel Dany. "Mindfulness Research and Applications in the Context of Neoliberalism: A Narrative and Critical Review." *Social and Personality Psychology Compass* 18, no. 2 (2024): e12936. https://doi.org/10.1111/spc3.12936.

The Chalkboard Editorial Team. "How Healthy Are Your Social Media Habits? 8 Tips To Upgrade Your Digital Wellness." *The Chalkboard* (blog), July 6, 2023. https://thechalkboardmag.com/healthy-social-media-habits/.

Chen, Kuan-Hsing, and David Morley, eds. *Stuart Hall: Critical Dialogues in Cultural Studies*. London: Routledge, 1996.

Chia, Aleena, Ana Jorge, and Tero Karppi, eds. *Reckoning with Social Media*. Lanham, MD: Rowman & Littlefield, 2021.

Christopher, John Chambers. "Situating Psychological Well-Being: Exploring the Cultural Roots of Its Theory and Research." *Journal of Counseling & Development* 77, no. 2 (1999): 141–52.

Chrulew, Matthew. "Pastoral Counter-conducts: Religious Resistance in Foucault's Genealogy of Christianity." *Critical Research on Religion* 2, no. 1 (2014): 55–65. https://doi.org/10.1177/2050303214520776.

Chun, Wendy Hui Kyong. *Updating to Remain the Same: Habitual New Media*. Cambridge, MA: MIT Press, 2017.

Citton, Yves. *The Ecology of Attention*. Translated by Barnaby Norman. Cambridge: Polity, 2017.

Cohen, Jason. "Tech Addiction Is Real: How to Cut Back on Screen Time and Wean Off Social Media." *PCMag UK*, May 12, 2023. https://uk.pcmag.com/ios/146827/tech-addiction-is-real-how-to-cut-back-on-screen-time-and-wean-off-social-media.

Coleman, James S. "Social Capital in the Creation of Human Capital." *American Journal of Sociology* 94 (1988): S95–120.

Coles-Brennan, Chantal, Anna Sulley, and Graeme Young. "Management of Digital Eye Strain." *Clinical and Experimental Optometry* 102, no. 1 (2019): 18–29. https://doi.org/10.1111/cxo.12798.

Collyer, Fran M. "Global Patterns in the Publishing of Academic Knowledge: Global North, Global South." *Current Sociology* 66, no. 1 (2018): 56–73. https://doi.org/10.1177/0011392116680020.

Cramer, Florian, and Matthew Fuller. "Interface." In *Software Studies: A Lexicon*, edited by Matthew Fuller. Cambridge, MA: MIT Press, 2008.

Cummins, Ian. "The Impact of Austerity on Mental Health Service Provision: A UK Perspective." *International Journal of Environmental Research and Public Health* 15, no. 6 (2018): 1145. https://doi.org/10.3390/ijerph15061145.

Cvetkovich, Ann. *Depression: A Public Feeling*. Durham, NC: Duke University Press, 2012.

Cyphers, Bennett, and Gennie Gebhart. "Behind the One-Way Mirror: A Deep Dive into the Technology of Corporate Surveillance." Electronic Frontier

Foundation, December 2, 2019. www.eff.org/wp/behind-the-one-way
-mirror.

Danziger, Kurt. *Constructing the Subject: Historical Origins of Psychological Research.* Cambridge: Cambridge University Press, 2009.

D'Arienzo, Maria Chiara, Valentina Boursier, and Mark D. Griffiths. "Addiction to Social Media and Attachment Styles: A Systematic Literature Review." *International Journal of Mental Health and Addiction* 17, no. 4 (2019): 1094–1118. https://doi.org/10.1007/s11469-019-00082-5.

Davidson, Arnold I. "In Praise of Counter-conduct." *History of the Human Sciences* 24, no. 4 (2011): 25–41. https://doi.org/10.1177/0952695111411625.

Davies, William. *The Happiness Industry: How the Government and Big Business Sold Us Well-Being.* London: Verso, 2015.

———. *The Limits of Neoliberalism: Authority, Sovereignty and the Logic of Competition.* London: SAGE, 2014.

Deacon, Roger. "Strategies of Governance Michel Foucault on Power." *Theoria: A Journal of Social and Political Theory*, no. 92 (1998): 113–48.

Dean, Mitchell M. *The Signature of Power: Sovereignty, Governmentality and Biopolitics.* London: SAGE, 2013.

Demetriou, Olga. "Counter-conduct and the Everyday: Anthropological Engagements with Philosophy." *Global Society* 30, no. 2 (2016): 218–37. https://doi.org/10.1080/13600826.2015.1133568.

Deville, Joe, Michael Guggenheim, and Zuzana Hrdličková. *Practising Comparison: Logics, Relations, Collaborations.* Manchester, UK: Mattering Press, 2016.

Dewey, John. *Human Nature and Conduct.* New York: Henry Holt, 1922.

Dijck, Jose van. "Datafication, Dataism and Dataveillance: Big Data between Scientific Paradigm and Ideology." *Surveillance & Society* 12, no. 2 (2014): 197–208. https://doi.org/10.24908/ss.v12i2.4776.

Dilts, Andrew. "From 'Entrepreneur of the Self' to 'Care of the Self': Neoliberal Governmentality and Foucault's Ethics." Paper presented at the Western Political Science Association 2010 Annual Meeting. https://papers.ssrn.com/abstract=1580709.

Docherty, Niall. "Facebook's Ideal User: Healthy Habits, Social Capital, and the Politics of Well-Being Online." *Social Media + Society* 6, no. 2 (2020): 2056305120915606. https://doi.org/10.1177/2056305120915606.

Dolata, Ulrich. "Privatization, Curation, Commodification." *Österreichische Zeitschrift für Soziologie* 44, no. 1 (2019): 181–97. https://doi.org/10.1007/s11614-019-00353-4.

Dorrestijn, Steven. "Technical Mediation and Subjectivation: Tracing and Extending Foucault's Philosophy of Technology." *Philosophy & Technology* 25, no. 2 (2012): 221–41, 236.

Dorrestijn, Steven, and Peter-Paul Verbeek. "Technology, Wellbeing, and Freedom: The Legacy of Utopian Design." *International Journal of Design* 7, no. 3 (2013): 45–56.

Drucker, Johanna. *Graphesis: Visual Forms of Knowledge Production.* Cambridge, MA: Harvard University Press, 2014.

Dyrberg, Torben Bech. "Foucault on Parrhesia: The Autonomy of Politics and Democracy." *Political Theory* 44, no. 2 (2016): 265–88. https://doi.org/10.1177/0090591715576082.

Egebark, Johan, and Mathias Ekström. "Can Indifference Make the World Greener?" *Journal of Environmental Economics and Management* 76 (March 2016): 1–13. https://doi.org/10.1016/j.jeem.2015.11.004.

Ekbia, Hamid, and Bonnie Nardi. "The Political Economy of Computing: The Elephant in the HCI Room." *Interactions* 22, no. 6 (2015): 46–49. https://doi.org/10.1145/2832117.

Ellison, Nicole B., Jessica Vitak, Rebecca Gray, and Cliff Lampe. "Cultivating Social Resources on Social Network Sites: Facebook Relationship Maintenance Behaviors and Their Role in Social Capital Processes." *Journal of Computer-Mediated Communication* 19, no. 4 (2014): 855–70.

Elmer, Greg. "Prospecting Facebook: The Limits of the Economy of Attention." *Media, Culture & Society* 41, no. 3 (2019): 332–46. https://doi.org/10.1177/0163443718813467.

Enli, Gunn, and Karin Fast. "Political Solutions or User Responsibilization? How Politicians Understand Problems Connected to Digital Overload." *Convergence* 29, no. 3 (2023): 675–89. https://doi.org/10.1177/13548565231160618.

Erfani, Seyedezahra Shadi, and Babak Abedin. "Impacts of the Use of Social Network Sites on Users' Psychological Well-Being: A Systematic Review." *Journal of the Association for Information Science and Technology* 69, no. 7 (2018): 900–12. https://doi.org/10.1002/asi.24015.

Eyal, Nir. *Hooked: How to Build Habit-Forming Products.* London: Penguin, 2014.

Falisi, Angela L., Kara P. Wiseman, Anna Gaysynsky, Jennifer K. Scheideler, Daniel A. Ramin, and Wen-ying Sylvia Chou. "Social Media for Breast Cancer Survivors: A Literature Review." *Journal of Cancer Survivorship* 11, no. 6 (2017): 808–21. https://doi.org/10.1007/s11764-017-0620-5.

Fallan, Kjetil. "De-scribing Design: Appropriating Script Analysis to Design History." *Design Issues* 24, no. 4 (2008): 61–75.

Fast, Karin. "The Disconnection Turn: Three Facets of Disconnective Work in Post-digital Capitalism." *Convergence* 27, no. 6 (2021): 1615–30. https://doi.org/10.1177/13548565211033382.

Feitsma, Joram, and Mark Whitehead. "Behavioural Expertise: Drift, Thrift and Shift under COVID-19." *International Review of Public Policy* 4, no. 2 (2022): 149–70. https://doi.org/10.4000/irpp.2634.

Ferragina, Emanuele, and Alessandro Arrigoni. "The Rise and Fall of Social Capital: Requiem for a Theory?" *Political Studies Review* 15, no. 3 (2017): 355–67. https://doi.org/10.1177/1478929915623968.

Fisher, Anthony L. "Social Media Is a Parasite, It Bleeds You to Live." *Business Insider*, September 6, 2020. www.businessinsider.com/delete-social-media-phone-parasite-mental-health-instagram-twitter-facebook-2020-9.

Fisher, Matthew. "A Theory of Public Wellbeing." *BMC Public Health* 19, no. 1 (2019): 1283. https://doi.org/10.1186/s12889-019-7626-z.

Fletcher, Guy. *The Routledge Handbook of Philosophy of Well-Being*. Routledge, 2015.

Fogg, B. J. *Persuasive Technology: Using Computers to Change What We Think and Do*. Boston: Morgan Kaufmann, 2003.

Foot, Philippa. *Natural Goodness*. Oxford: Clarendon Press, 2001.

Fornet-Betancourt, Raúl, Helmut Becker, Alfredo Gomez-Müller, and J. D. Dauthier. "The Ethic of Care for the Self as a Practice of Freedom: An Interview with Michel Foucault on January 20, 1984." *Philosophy & Social Criticism* 12, no. 2–3 (1987): 112–31. https://doi.org/10.1177/019145378701200202.

Foucault, Michel. *Archaeology of Knowledge*. New York: Routledge, 2002.

———. *The Birth of Biopolitics: Lectures at the Collège de France, 1978–79*. Basingstoke, UK: Palgrave Macmillan, 2010.

———. *Discipline and Punish: The Birth of the Prison*. New York: Vintage Books, 1995.

———. *Ethics: Subjectivity and Truth (The Essential Works of Foucault, 1954–1984, vol. 1)*, edited by Paul Rabinow. New York: The New Press, 1997.

———. *The Hermeneutics of the Subject: Lectures at the Collège de France 1981–1982*. New York: Picador, 2005.

———. *The History of Sexuality, vol. 1: An Introduction*. London: Penguin, 1998.

———. *The History of Sexuality, vol. 2: The Use of Pleasure*. New York: Vintage Books, 1990.

———. "Is It Really Important to Think? An Interview Translated by Thomas Keenan." *Philosophy & Social Criticism* 9, no. 1 (1982): 30–40. https://doi.org/10.1177/019145378200900102.

———. "The Lives of Infamous Men." In *Power (The Essential Works of Foucault, 1954–1984, vol. 3)*, edited by James D. Faubion, translated by Robert Hurley. New York: The New Press, 2001.

———. "Nietzsche, Genealogy, History." In *Language, Counter-memory, Practice: Selected Essays and Interviews*, edited by Donald F. Bouchard, 139–65. Ithaca, NY: Cornell University Press, 2019.

———. *On the Government of the Living: Lectures at the Collège de France, 1979–1980*. New York: Picador, 2016.

———. *The Politics of Truth*. Edited by Sylvère Lotringer. Los Angeles: Semiotext(e), 2007.

———. *The Punitive Society: Lectures at the Collège de France, 1972–1973*. Edited by Arnold I. Davidson. Translated by Graham Burchell. New York: Palgrave Macmillan, 2015.

———. *Security, Territory, Population: Lectures at the Collège de France, 1977–78*. Basingstoke, UK: Palgrave Macmillan, 2007.

———. "The Subject and Power." In Hubert L. Dreyfus and Paul Rabinow, *Michel Foucault: Beyond Structuralism and Hermeneutics*, 208–29. Chicago: University of Chicago Press, 1983.

Foucault, Michel, and Graham Burchell. "Parrēsia." *Critical Inquiry* 41, no. 2 (2015): 219–53. https://doi.org/10.1086/679075.

Foucault, Michel, and Colin Gordon. *Power/Knowledge: Selected Interviews and Other Writings, 1972–1977*. New York: Pantheon Books, 1980.

Foucault, Michel, Luther H. Martin, Huck Gutman, and Patrick H. Hutton, eds. *Technologies of the Self: A Seminar with Michel Foucault*. Amherst: University of Massachusetts Press, 1988.

Fraser, Nancy. "Foucault on Modern Power: Empirical Insights and Normative Confusions." *Praxis International* 1, no. 3 (1981): 272–87.

Fraser, Nancy, and Rahel Jaeggi. *Capitalism: A Conversation in Critical Theory*. Cambridge: Polity, 2018.

Friedman, Milton, and Rose Friedman. *Free to Choose: A Personal Statement*. New York: Harcourt Brace Jovanovich, 1990.

Fuchs, Christian. *Culture and Economy in the Age of Social Media*. New York: Routledge, 2015.

———. "Digital Prosumption Labour on Social Media in the Context of the Capitalist Regime of Time." *Time & Society* 23, no. 1 (2014): 97–123. https://doi.org/10.1177/0961463X13502117.

Fuller, Matthew, and Andrew Goffey. *Evil Media*. Cambridge, MA: MIT Press, 2012.

Gadelrab, Sherry Sayed. "Medical Healers in Ottoman Egypt, 1517–1805." *Medical History* 54, no. 3 (2010): 365–86. https://doi.org/10.1017/S0025727300004658.

Galea, Sandro, Monica Uddin, and Karestan Koenen. "The Urban Environment and Mental Disorders." *Epigenetics* 6, no. 4 (2011): 400–4. https://doi.org/10.4161/epi.6.4.14944.

Galloway, Alexander R. *The Interface Effect*. Cambridge: Polity, 2012.

Gamby, Katie, Dominique Burns, and Kaitlyn Forristal. "Wellness Decolonized: The History of Wellness and Recommendations for the Counseling Field." *Journal of Mental Health Counseling* 43, no. 3 (2021): 228–45. https://doi.org/10.17744/mehc.43.3.05.

Gerlitz, Carolin, and Anne Helmond. "The Like Economy: Social Buttons and the Data-Intensive Web." *New Media & Society* 15, no. 8 (2013): 1348–65. https://doi.org/10.1177/1461444812472322.

Gershon, Ilana. "'Neoliberal Agency.'" *Current Anthropology* 52, no. 4 (2011): 537–55. https://doi.org/10.1086/660866.

———. "Publish and Be Damned: New Media Publics and Neoliberal Risk." *Ethnography* 15, no. 1 (2014): 70–87. https://doi.org/10.1177/1466138113502514.

———. "Un-Friend My Heart: Facebook, Promiscuity, and Heartbreak in a Neoliberal Age." *Anthropological Quarterly* 84, no. 4 (2011): 865–94.

Ghaffari, Soudeh. "Discourses of Celebrities on Instagram: Digital Femininity, Self-Representation and Hate Speech." *Critical Discourse Studies* 19, no. 2 (2022): 161–78. https://doi.org/10.1080/17405904.2020.1839923.

Ghai, Sakshi, Lucía Magis-Weinberg, Mariya Stoilova, Sonia Livingstone, and Amy Orben. "Social Media and Adolescent Well-Being in the Global South." *Current Opinion in Psychology* 46 (August 2022): 101318. https://doi.org/10.1016/j.copsyc.2022.101318.

Gibson, Anna D., Niall Docherty, and Tarleton Gillespie. "Health and Toxicity in Content Moderation: The Discursive Work of Justification." *Information, Communication & Society* 27, no. 7 (2024): 1441–57. https://doi.org/10.1080/1369118X.2023.2291456.

Gigerenzer, Gerd. "On the Supposed Evidence for Libertarian Paternalism." *Review of Philosophy and Psychology* 6, no. 3 (2015): 361–83. https://doi.org/10.1007/s13164-015-0248-1.

Gillespie, Tarleton. *Custodians of the Internet: Platforms, Content Moderation, and the Hidden Decisions That Shape Social Media*. New Haven, CT: Yale University Press, 2018.

———. "The Fact of Content Moderation; or, Let's Not Solve the Platforms' Problems for Them." *Media and Communication* 11, no. 2 (2023). https://doi.org/10.17645/mac.v11i2.6610.

Golder, Ben. *Foucault and the Politics of Rights*. Stanford, CA: Stanford University Press, 2015.

GOV.UK. "UK CMO Commentary on Screen Time and Social Media Map of Reviews." Department of Health and Social Care, February 7, 2019. www.gov.uk/government/publications/uk-cmo-commentary-on-screen-time-and-social-media-map-of-reviews.

Gramsci, Antonio. *The Modern Prince and Other Writings*. Reprint edition. New York: International Publishers, 1959.

Granovetter, Mark S. "The Strength of Weak Ties." *American Journal of Sociology* 78, no. 6 (1973): 1360–80.

Gray, Colin M., Yubo Kou, Bryan Battles, Joseph Hoggatt, and Austin L. Toombs. "The Dark (Patterns) Side of UX Design." In *CHI '18: Proceedings of the 2018 CHI Conference on Human Factors in Computing Systems*, 1–14 New York: Association for Computing Machinery, 2018. https://doi.org/10.1145/3173574.3174108.

Greenhalgh, Trisha, and Simon Wessely. "'Health for Me': A Sociocultural Analysis of Healthism in the Middle Classes." *British Medical Bulletin* 69 (2004): 197–213. https://doi.org/10.1093/bmb/ldh013.

Greenstone, Gerry. "The History of Bloodletting." *BC Medical Journal* 52, no. 1 (2010): 12–14.

Grosser, Benjamin. "What Do Metrics Want? How Quantification Prescribes Social Interaction on Facebook." *Computational Culture*, no. 4 (November 9, 2014). http://computationalculture.net/what-do-metrics-want/.

Guan, Xiaofei, Guoxin Fan, Zhengqi Chen, Ying Zeng, Hailong Zhang, Annan Hu, Guangfei Gu, Xinbo Wu, Xin Gu, and Shisheng He. "Gender Difference in Mobile Phone Use and the Impact of Digital Device Exposure on Neck Posture." *Ergonomics* 59, no. 11 (2016): 1453–61. https://doi.org/10.1080/00140139.2016.1147614.

The Guardian Live. "Mark Zuckerberg Testifies before Congress—Watch Live," streamed on YouTube, April 10, 2018. www.youtube.com/watch?v=mZaec_mlq9M.

Guthman, Julie. *Weighing In: Obesity, Food Justice, and the Limits of Capitalism*. Berkeley: University of California Press, 2011.

Habermas, Jürgen, and Seyla Ben-Habib. "Modernity versus Postmodernity." *New German Critique*, no. 22 (1981): 3–14. https://doi.org/10.2307/487859.

Hadler, Florian, and Joachim Haupt, eds. "Towards a Critique of Interfaces." In *Interface Critique*, 7–13. Berlin: Kulturverlag Kadmos, 2016.

Haidt, Jonathan. *The Anxious Generation: How the Great Rewiring of Childhood Is Causing an Epidemic of Mental Illness*. London: Penguin, 2024.

Halpern, David. *Inside the Nudge Unit: How Small Changes Can Make a Big Difference*. London: W. H. Allen, 2015.

Hamann, Trent H. "Neoliberalism, Governmentality, and Ethics." *Foucault Studies*, no. 6 (February 2009): 37–59. https://doi.org/10.22439/fs.v0i0.2471.

Hanlon, Gerard, and Peter Fleming. "Updating the Critical Perspective on Corporate Social Responsibility." *Sociology Compass* 3, no. 6 (2009): 937–48. https://doi.org/10.1111/j.1751-9020.2009.00250.x.

Harsin, Jayson. "Regimes of Posttruth, Postpolitics, and Attention Economies." *Communication, Culture and Critique* 8, no. 2 (2015): 327–33. https://doi.org/10.1111/cccr.12097.

Harvey, David. *A Brief History of Neoliberalism*. Oxford: Oxford University Press, 2005.

Hillis, Ken, Susanna Paasonen, and Michael Petit, eds. *Networked Affect*. Cambridge, MA: MIT Press, 2015.

Hoang, Quynh, James Cronin, and Alexandros Skandalis. "Futureless Vicissitudes: Gestural Anti-consumption and the Reflexively Impotent (Anti-)consumer." *Marketing Theory* 23, no. 4 (2023). https://doi.org/10.1177/14705931231153193.

Hobart, Hi'ilei Julia Kawehipuaakahaopulani, and Tamara Kneese. "Radical Care." *Social Text* 38, no. 1 (2020): 1–16. https://doi.org/10.1215/01642472-7971067.

Hoffner, Cynthia A., and Bradley J. Bond. "Parasocial Relationships, Social Media, & Well-Being." *Current Opinion in Psychology* 45 (June 2022): 101306. https://doi.org/10.1016/j.copsyc.2022.101306.

Hookway, Branden. *Interface*. Cambridge, MA: MIT Press, 2014.

Howard, Lindsay M., Kristin E. Heron, Rachel I. MacIntyre, Taryn A. Myers, and Robin S. Everhart. "Is Use of Social Networking Sites Associated with Young Women's Body Dissatisfaction and Disordered Eating? A Look at Black-White Racial Differences." *Body Image* 23 (December 2017): 109–13. https://doi.org/10.1016/j.bodyim.2017.08.008.

Humphreys, Lee. *The Qualified Self: Social Media and the Accounting of Everyday Life*. Cambridge, MA: MIT Press, 2018.

Ingram, David, ed. *The Political*. Malden, MA: Blackwell, 2002.

Ishikawa, Maria. "Mindfulness in Western Contexts Perpetuates Oppressive Realities for Minority Cultures: The Consequences of Cultural Appropriation." *SFU Educational Review* 11, no. 1 (2018). https://doi.org/10.21810/sfuer.v11i1.757.

Isin, Engin F. "The Neurotic Citizen." *Citizenship Studies* 8, no. 3 (2004): 217–35.

Islam, M. Mofizul. "Social Determinants of Health and Related Inequalities: Confusion and Implications." *Frontiers in Public Health* 7 (February 2019): article 11. https://doi.org/10.3389/fpubh.2019.00011.

Jablonsky, Rebecca. "Meditation Apps and the Promise of Attention by Design." *Science, Technology, & Human Values* 47, no. 2 (2022): 314–36. https://doi.org/10.1177/01622439211049276.

Jaeggi, Rahel. *Critique of Forms of Life*. Cambridge, MA: Belknap Press of Harvard University Press, 2018.

Jasanoff, Sheila, and Sang-Hyun Kim, eds. *Dreamscapes of Modernity: Sociotechnical Imaginaries and the Fabrication of Power*. Chicago: University of Chicago Press, 2015.

Jorge, Ana. "Social Media, Interrupted: Users Recounting Temporary Disconnection on Instagram." *Social Media + Society* 5, no. 4 (2019): https://doi.org/10.1177/2056305119881691.

Jorge, Ana, Inês Amaral, and Artur de Matos Alves. "'Time Well Spent': The Ideology of Temporal Disconnection as a Means for Digital Well-Being." *International Journal of Communication* 16 (2022): 1551–72.

Jørgensen, Kristian Møller. "The Media Go-Along: Researching Mobilities with Media at Hand." *MedieKultur: Journal of Media and Communication Research* 32, no. 60 (2016). https://doi.org/10.7146/mediekultur.v32i60.22429.

Jupp, Eleanor, Jessica Pykett, and Fiona Smith, eds. *Emotional States: Sites and Spaces of Affective Governance*. New York: Routledge, 2017.

Kahneman, Daniel. *Thinking, Fast and Slow*. London: Penguin Books, 2012.

Kaiser, Bonnie N., and Lesley Jo Weaver. "Culture-Bound Syndromes, Idioms of Distress, and Cultural Concepts of Distress: New Directions for an Old Concept in Psychological Anthropology." *Transcultural Psychiatry* 56, no. 4 (2019): 589–98. https://doi.org/10.1177/1363461519862708.

Kant, Immanuel. "An Answer to the Question: What Is Enlightenment? (1784)." In *Practical Philosophy*, edited by Mary J. Gregor, 11–22. Cambridge: Cambridge University Press, 1996.

Kaplan, Jonathan. "Self-Care as Self-Blame Redux: Stress as Personal and Political." *Kennedy Institute of Ethics Journal* 29, no. 2 (2019): 97–123. https://doi.org/10.1353/ken.2019.0017.

Karim, Fazida, Azeezat Oyewande, Lamis F. Abdalla, Reem Chaudhry Ehsanullah, and Safeera Khan. "Social Media Use and Its Connection to Mental Health: A Systematic Review." *Cureus*, June 15, 2020. https://doi.org /10.7759/cureus.8627.

Karppi, Tero. *Disconnect: Facebook's Affective Bonds*. Minneapolis: University of Minnesota Press, 2018.

Kaun, Anne. "Ways of Seeing Digital Disconnection: A Negative Sociology of Digital Culture." *Convergence* 27, no. 6 (2021): 1571–83.

Kaye, Linda K., Amy Orben, David A. Ellis, Simon C. Hunter, and Stephen Houghton. "The Conceptual and Methodological Mayhem of 'Screen Time.'" *International Journal of Environmental Research and Public Health* 17, no. 10 (2020): 3661. https://doi.org/10.3390/ijerph17103661.

Keating, Lydia. "I'm an Influencer, and I Think Social Media Is Toxic." *Slate*, February 1, 2022. https://slate.com/technology/2022/02/instagram-tiktok-influencer-social-media-dangers.html.

Keles, Betul, Niall McCrae, and Annmarie Grealish. "A Systematic Review: The Influence of Social Media on Depression, Anxiety and Psychological Distress in Adolescents." *International Journal of Adolescence and Youth* 25, no. 1 (2020): 79–93. https://doi.org/10.1080/02673843.2019.1590851.

Klein, Elise, China Mills, Asha Achuthan, and Eva Hilberg. "Human Technologies, Affect and the Global Psy-Complex." *Economy and Society* 50, no. 3 (2021): 347–58. https://doi.org/10.1080/03085147.2021.1899658.

Kross, Ethan, Philippe Verduyn, Gal Sheppes, Cory K. Costello, John Jonides, and Oscar Ybarra. "Social Media and Well-Being: Pitfalls, Progress, and Next Steps." *Trends in Cognitive Sciences* 25, no. 1 (2021): 55–66.

Lacey, Cherie, Alex Beattie, and Catherine Caudwell. "Wellness Capitalism and the Design of the Perfect User." *Interface Critique* 3 (2021): 127–50. https:// doi.org/10.11588/IC.2021.3.81323.

Langlois, Ganaele, and Greg Elmer. "The Research Politics of Social Media Platforms." *Culture Machine* 14 (2013). www.academia.edu/download /31951866/505-1170-1-PB_(1).pdf.

Latour, Bruno. "On Technical Mediation." *Common Knowledge* 3, no. 2 (1994): 29–64.

———. *Reassembling the Social: An Introduction to Actor-Network-Theory*. Oxford: Oxford University Press, 2005.

———. "Where Are the Missing Masses? The Sociology of a Few Mundane Artifacts." *Shaping Technology/Building Society: Studies in Sociotechnical Change* 1 (1992): 225–58.

Lee, Hae Yeon, Jeremy P. Jamieson, Harry T. Reis, Christopher G. Beevers, Robert A. Josephs, Michael C. Mullarkey, Joseph M. O'Brien, and David S. Yeager. "Getting Fewer 'Likes' Than Others on Social Media Elicits Emotional Distress among Victimized Adolescents." *Child Development* 91, no. 6 (2020): 2141–59. https://doi.org/10.1111/cdev.13422.

Lee, Min Kyung, Sara Kiesler, and Jodi Forlizzi. "Mining Behavioral Economics to Design Persuasive Technology for Healthy Choices." In *CHI '11: Proceedings of the Sigchi Conference on Human Factors in Computing Systems*, 325–34. New York: Association for Computing Machinery, 2011.

Leerssen, Paddy. "Outside the Black Box: From Algorithmic Transparency to Platform Observability in the Digital Services Act." *Weizenbaum Journal of the Digital Society* 4, no. 2 (2024). https://doi.org/10.34669/wi.wjds/4.2.3.

Leggett, Will. "The Politics of Behaviour Change: Nudge, Neoliberalism and the State." *Policy & Politics* 42, no. 1 (2014): 3–19. https://doi.org/10.1332/030557312X655576.

Lemke, Thomas. "Critique and Experience in Foucault." *Theory, Culture & Society* 28, no. 4 (2011): 26–48. https://doi.org/10.1177/0263276411404907.

———. *Foucault, Governmentality, and Critique*. New York: Routledge, 2015.

Light, Ben, Jean Burgess, and Stefanie Duguay. "The Walkthrough Method: An Approach to the Study of Apps." *New Media & Society* 20, no. 3 (2018): 881–900. https://doi.org/10.1177/1461444816675438.

Lim, Sungju, Dumebi Nzegwu, and Michelle L. Wright. "The Impact of Psychosocial Stress from Life Trauma and Racial Discrimination on Epigenetic Aging—a Systematic Review." *Biological Research for Nursing* 24, no. 2 (2022): 202–15. https://doi.org/10.1177/10998004211060561.

Little, Nicolette. "Social Media 'Ghosts': How Facebook (Meta) Memories Complicates Healing for Survivors of Intimate Partner Violence." *Feminist Media Studies* 23, no. 8 (2023): 1–23. https://doi.org/10.1080/14680777.2022.2149593.

Littler, Jo. *Against Meritocracy: Culture, Power and Myths of Mobility*. London: Routledge, 2017.

Locke, Abigail, Rebecca Lawthom, and Antonia Lyons. "Social Media Platforms as Complex and Contradictory Spaces for Feminisms: Visibility, Opportunity, Power, Resistance and Activism." *Feminism & Psychology* 28, no. 1 (2018): 3–10. https://doi.org/10.1177/0959353517753973.

Lorde, Audre, and Sonia Sanchez. *A Burst of Light: And Other Essays*. Garden City, NY: Ixia Press, 2017.

Lorenzini, Daniele. "From Counter-conduct to Critical Attitude: Michel Foucault and the Art of Not Being Governed Quite So Much." *Foucault Studies*, no. 21 (June 28 2016): 7–21. https://doi.org/10.22439/fs.v0i0.5011.

Lupton, Deborah. *Fat*. Second edition. London: Routledge, 2018.

Maaranen, Anna, and Janne Tienari. "Social Media and Hyper-masculine Work Cultures." *Gender, Work & Organization* 27, no. 6 (2020): 1127–44. https://doi.org/10.1111/gwao.12450.

Manovich, Lev. *The Language of New Media*. Cambridge, MA: MIT Press, 2001.

Marmot, Michael, and Richard Wilkinson. *Social Determinants of Health*. Oxford: Oxford University Press, 2005.

Marshall, Matt. "Facebook Launches 'News Feed' and 'Mini Feed'—as YouTube Invades Turf." *VentureBeat* (blog), September 5, 2006. https://venturebeat.com/business/facebook-launches-news-feed-and-mini-feed-as-youtube-invades-turf/.

Marwick, Alice E. "The Public Domain: Surveillance in Everyday Life." *Surveillance & Society* 9, no. 4 (2012): 378–93. https://doi.org/10.24908/ss.v9i4.4342.

Marwick, Alice E., and danah boyd. "I Tweet Honestly, I Tweet Passionately: Twitter Users, Context Collapse, and the Imagined Audience." *New Media & Society* 13, no. 1 (2011): 114–33. https://doi.org/10.1177/1461444810365313.

Marx, Karl, and Frederick Engels. *Economic and Philosophic Manuscripts of 1844*. Translated by Martin Milligan. Radford, VA: Wilder, 2011.

Marya, Rupa, and Raj Patel. *Inflamed: Deep Medicine and the Anatomy of Injustice*. London: Allen Lane, 2021.

McGuigan, Jim. *Neoliberal Culture*. Basingstoke, UK: Palgrave Macmillan, 2016.

McLean, Chris, and John Hassard. "Symmetrical Absence/Symmetrical Absurdity: Critical Notes on the Production of Actor-Network Accounts." *Journal of Management Studies* 41, no. 3 (2004): 493–519. https://doi.org/10.1111/j.1467-6486.2004.00442.x.

Meier, Adrian, Alicia Gilbert, Sophie Börner, and Daniel Possler. "Instagram Inspiration: How Upward Comparison on Social Network Sites Can Contribute to Well-Being." *Journal of Communication* 70, no. 5 (2020): 721–43. https://doi.org/10.1093/joc/jqaa025.

Meier, Adrian, and Benjamin K. Johnson. "Social Comparison and Envy on Social Media: A Critical Review." *Current Opinion in Psychology* 45 (June 2022): 101302. https://doi.org/10.1016/j.copsyc.2022.101302.

Meier, Adrian, and Leonard Reinecke. "Computer-Mediated Communication, Social Media, and Mental Health: A Conceptual and Empirical Meta-Review." *Communication Research* 48, no. 8 (2021): 1182–1209. https://doi.org/10.1177/0093650220958224.

Meta. "Bringing People Closer Together," January 12, 2018. https://about.fb.com/news/2018/01/news-feed-fyi-bringing-people-closer-together/.

———. "Building a Better News Feed for You," June 29, 2016. https://about.fb.com/news/2016/06/building-a-better-news-feed-for-you/.

———. "Facebook Launches Additional Privacy Controls for News Feed and Mini-Feed," September 8, 2006. https://about.fb.com/news/2006/09/facebook-launches-additional-privacy-controls-for-news-feed-and-mini-feed/.

———. "Hard Questions: Is Spending Time on Social Media Bad for Us?," December 15, 2017. https://about.fb.com/news/2017/12/hard-questions-is-spending-time-on-social-media-bad-for-us/.

———. "Health & Well-Being—Digital Wellness." Accessed June 1, 2023. https://about.meta.com/actions/safety/topics/wellbeing/digitalwellness/.

———. "Health & Well-Being—Youth Well-Being." Accessed February 6, 2024. https://about.meta.com/actions/safety/audiences/youth/health-well-being/.

———. "How Feed Works." Facebook Help Center. Accessed September 19, 2023. www.facebook.com/help/1155510281178725/?helpref=hc_fnav.

———. "Introducing Hard Questions," June 15, 2017. https://about.fb.com/news/2017/06/hard-questions/.

———. "Like and React to Posts." Facebook Help Center. Accessed September 19, 2023. www.facebook.com/help/1624177224568554?helpref=hc_fnav.

———. "Making News Feed an Easier Place to Connect and Navigate," August 15, 2017. https://about.fb.com/news/2017/08/making-news-feed-an-easier-place-to-connect-and-navigate/.

Meta for Developers. "Meta for Developers—From Consumption to Connection." Accessed August 24, 2023. https://developers.facebook.com/videos/f8-2018/from-consumption-to-connection/.

Miller, Boaz. "Is Technology Value-Neutral?" *Science, Technology, & Human Values* 46, no. 1 (2021): 53–80. https://doi.org/10.1177/0162243919900965.

Miller, Peter, and Nikolas Rose. *Governing the Present: Administering Economic, Social and Personal Life.* Cambridge: Polity, 2008.

Milner, Andrew. "Cultural Materialism, Culturalism and Post-culturalism: The Legacy of Raymond Williams." *Theory, Culture & Society* 11, no. 1 (1994): 43–73. https://doi.org/10.1177/026327694011001005.

Mirowski, Philip. *Never Let a Serious Crisis Go to Waste: How Neoliberalism Survived the Financial Meltdown.* London: Verso, 2014.

Morgans, Julian. "The Inventor of the 'Like' Button Wants You to Stop Worrying about Likes." *Vice* (blog), July 6, 2017. www.vice.com/en/article/mbag3a /the-inventor-of-the-like-button-wants-you-to-stop-worrying-about-likes.

Murphy, Michelle. *The Economization of Life.* Durham, NC: Duke University Press, 2017.

Natale, Simone, and Emiliano Treré. "Vinyl Won't Save Us: Reframing Disconnection as Engagement." *Media, Culture & Society* 42, no. 4 (2020): 626–33. https://doi.org/10.1177/0163443720914027.

Neff, Gina, and Dawn Nafus. *Self-Tracking.* Cambridge, MA: MIT Press, 2016.

Nelson, Lisa S. *Social Media and Morality: Losing Our Self Control.* Cambridge: Cambridge University Press, 2018.

Nestler, Eric J., Catherine J. Peña, Marija Kundakovic, Amanda Mitchell, and Schahram Akbarian. "Epigenetic Basis of Mental Illness." *The Neuroscientist* 22, no. 5 (2016): 447–63. https://doi.org/10.1177/1073858415608147.

Neupane, Aatish, Derek Hansen, Anud Sharma, Jerry Alan Fails, Bikalpa Neupane, and Jeremy Beutler. "A Review of Gamified Fitness Tracker Apps and Future Directions." In *CHI PLAY '20: Proceedings of the Annual Symposium on Computer-Human Interaction in Play.* 522–33. New York: Association for Computing Machinery, 2020.

Newall, Philip W. S., Leonardo Weiss-Cohen, Henrik Singmann, Lukasz Walasek, and Elliot A Ludvig. "Impact of the 'When the Fun Stops, Stop' Gambling Message on Online Gambling Behaviour: A Randomised, Online Experimental Study." *The Lancet Public Health* 7, no. 5 (2022): e437–46. https://doi.org/10.1016/S2468-2667(21)00279-6.

Ng, Aik Kwang, David Y. F. Ho, Shyh Shin Wong, and Ian Smith. "In Search of the Good Life: A Cultural Odyssey in the East and West." *Genetic, Social, and General Psychology Monographs* 129, no. 4 (2003): 317–63.

Ngai, Sianne. *Ugly Feelings.* Cambridge, MA: Harvard University Press, 2007.

NHS. "Live Well," January 17, 2022. www.nhs.uk/live-well/.

Nichter, Mark. "Idioms of Distress: Alternatives in the Expression of Psychosocial Distress: A Case Study from South India." *Culture, Medicine and Psychiatry* 5, no. 4 (1981): 379–408. https://doi.org/10.1007/BF00054782.

———. "Idioms of Distress Revisited." *Culture, Medicine, and Psychiatry* 34, no. 2 (2010): 401–16. https://doi.org/10.1007/s11013-010-9179-6.

Nietzsche, Friedrich. *On the Genealogy of Morals: A Polemic.* Translated by Michael A. Scarpitti. London: Penguin Books, 2013.

NIH News in Health. "Healthy Social Media Habits." September 2022. https://newsinhealth.nih.gov/2022/09/healthy-social-media-habits.

Nissenbaum, Helen. "From Preemption to Circumvention: If Technology Regulates, Why Do We Need Regulation (and Vice Versa)." *Berkeley Technology Law Journal* 26 (2011): 1367–86.

O'Day, Emily B., and Richard G. Heimberg. "Social Media Use, Social Anxiety, and Loneliness: A Systematic Review." *Computers in Human Behavior Reports* 3 (2021): 100070.

Oliver, Mary Beth. "Social Media Use and Eudaimonic Well-Being." *Current Opinion in Psychology* 45 (June 2022): 101307. https://doi.org/10.1016/j.copsyc.2022.101307.

Olivier, Bert. "Capitalism and Suffering." *Psychology in Society*, no. 48 (2015): 1–21. https://doi.org/10.17159/2309-8708/2015/n48a1.

Oman, Susan. *Understanding Well-Being Data: Improving Social and Cultural Policy, Practice and Research.* Cham, Switzerland: Palgrave Macmillan, 2021.

Orlowski-Yang, Jeff, dir. *The Social Dilemma.* Film. Boulder, CO: Exposure Labs, Argent Pictures, The Space Program, 2020.

Oudshoorn, Nelly, and Trevor Pinch, eds. *How Users Matter: The Co-construction of Users and Technology.* Cambridge, MA: MIT Press, 2003.

Ovide, Shira. "Are You Mindlessly Scrolling? Here's How to Tame Your Bad Tech Habit." *The Washington Post,* March 7, 2023. www.washingtonpost.com/technology/2023/03/07/taming-bad-tech-habbit/.

Papacharissi, Zizi, Thomas Streeter, and Tarleton Gillespie. "Culture Digitally: Habitus of the New." *Journal of Broadcasting & Electronic Media* 57, no. 4 (2013): 596–607. https://doi.org/10.1080/08838151.2013.846344.

Peake, Jonathan M., Graham Kerr, and John P. Sullivan. "A Critical Review of Consumer Wearables, Mobile Applications, and Equipment for Providing Biofeedback, Monitoring Stress, and Sleep in Physically Active Populations." *Frontiers in Physiology* 9 (2018). www.frontiersin.org/articles/10.3389/fphys.2018.00743.

Peck, Jamie. *Constructions of Neoliberal Reason.* Oxford: Oxford University Press, 2010.

Pedersen, Morten Axel, Kristoffer Albris, and Nick Seaver. "The Political Economy of Attention." *Annual Review of Anthropology* 50, no. 1 (2021): 309–25. https://doi.org/10.1146/annurev-anthro-101819-110356.

Pedwell, Carolyn. "Habit and the Politics of Social Change: A Comparison of Nudge Theory and Pragmatist Philosophy." *Body & Society* 23, no. 4 (2017): 59–94. https://doi.org/10.1177/1357034X17734619.

Pfaffenberger, Bryan. "Technological Dramas." *Science, Technology, & Human Values* 17, no. 3 (1992): 282–312. https://doi.org/10.1177/016224399201700302.

Pichert, Daniel, and Konstantinos V. Katsikopoulos. "Green Defaults: Information Presentation and pro-Environmental Behaviour." *Journal of Environmental Psychology* 28, no. 1 (2008): 63–73. https://doi.org/10.1016/j.jenvp.2007.09.004.

Pilkington, Marc. "Well-Being, Happiness and the Structural Crisis of Neoliberalism: An Interdisciplinary Analysis through the Lenses of Emotions." *Mind & Society* 15, no. 2 (2016): 265–80. https://doi.org/10.1007/s11299-015-0181-0.

Portwood-Stacer, Laura. "Media Refusal and Conspicuous Non-consumption: The Performative and Political Dimensions of Facebook Abstention." *New Media & Society* 15, no. 7 (2013): 1041–57. https://doi.org/10.1177/1461444812465139.

Pötzsch, Holger. "Critical Digital Literacy: Technology in Education beyond Issues of User Competence and Labour-Market Qualifications." *tripleC: Communication, Capitalism & Critique* 17, no. 2 (2019): 221–40. https://doi.org/10.31269/triplec.v17i2.1093.

Pultz, Sabina. "Shame and Passion: The Affective Governing of Young Unemployed People." *Theory & Psychology* 28, no. 3 (2018): 358–81. https://doi.org/10.1177/0959354318759608.

Quijano, Aníbal. "Coloniality of Power and Eurocentrism in Latin America." *International Sociology* 15, no. 2 (2000): 215–32. https://doi.org/10.1177/0268580900015002005.

Rabinow, Paul. *Anthropos Today: Reflections on Modern Equipment*. Princeton, NJ: Princeton University Press, 2003.

Raibley, Jason. "Health and Well-Being." *Philosophical Studies* 165 (2013): 469–89.

Rajchman, John. "Ethics after Foucault." *Social Text*, no. 13/14 (1986): 165–83.

Rebonato, Riccardo. "A Critical Assessment of Libertarian Paternalism." *Journal of Consumer Policy* 37, no. 3 (2014): 357–96. https://doi.org/10.1007/s10603-014-9265-1.

Redström, Johan. "Persuasive Design: Fringes and Foundations." In *Persuasive Technology*, edited by Wijnand A. IJsselsteijn, Yvonne A.W. de Kort, Cees Midden, Berry Eggen, and Elise van den Hoven, 112–22. Berlin: Springer, 2006.

Reinecke, Leonard, Christoph Klimmt, Adrian Meier, Sabine Reich, Dorothée Hefner, Katharina Knop-Huelss, Diana Rieger, and Peter Vorderer. "Permanently Online and Permanently Connected: Development and

Validation of the Online Vigilance Scale." *PLoS One* 13, no. 10 (2018): e0205384. https://doi.org/10.1371/journal.pone.0205384.

Reinecke, Leonard, and Adrian Meier. "Guilt and Media Use." In *The International Encyclopedia of Media Psychology*, edited by Jan van den Bulck and David R. Roskos-Ewoldsen. London: Wiley, 2020.

Reuters. "Facebook Will Try to 'Nudge' Teens Away from Harmful Content." October 10, 2021. www.reuters.com/technology/facebook-will-try-nudge -teens-away-harmful-content-2021-10-10/.

Robards, Brady, and Siân Lincoln. "Uncovering Longitudinal Life Narratives: Scrolling Back on Facebook." *Qualitative Research* 17, no. 6 (2017): 715–30. https://doi.org/10.1177/1468794117700707.

Roberts, John M., and Colin Cremin. "Prosumer Culture and the Question of Fetishism." *Journal of Consumer Culture* 19, no. 2 (2019): 213–30. https:// doi.org/10.1177/1469540517717773.

Roberts, Sam G. B., and Robin I. M. Dunbar. "Communication in Social Networks: Effects of Kinship, Network Size, and Emotional Closeness." *Personal Relationships* 18, no. 3 (2011): 439–52. https://doi.org/10.1111/j .1475-6811.2010.01310.x.

Roffarello, Alberto Monge, Luigi De Russis, Danielle Lottridge, and Marta E. Cecchinato. "Understanding Digital Wellbeing within Complex Technological Contexts." *International Journal of Human-Computer Studies* 175 (July 2023): 103034. https://doi.org/10.1016/j.ijhcs.2023.103034.

Rommes, E. W. M. "Gender Scripts and the Internet: The Design and Use of Amserdam's [*sic*] Digital City." PhD diss., University of Twente, 2002. https:// research.utwente.nl/en/publications/gender-scripts-and-the-internet-the -design-and-use-of-amserdams-d.

Rorty, Amélie, and James Schmidt. *Kant's Idea for a Universal History with a Cosmopolitan Aim: A Critical Guide*. Cambridge: Cambridge University Press, 2009.

Rose, Nikolas. *Governing the Soul: Shaping of the Private Self*. Second edition. London: Free Association Books, 1999.

———. *Inventing Our Selves: Psychology, Power, and Personhood*, revised edition. Cambridge: Cambridge University Press, 2010.

———. *Politics of Life Itself: Biomedicine, Power, and Subjectivity in the Twenty-First Century*. Princeton, NJ: Princeton University Press, 2007.

———. *The Psychological Complex: Psychology, Politics, and Society in England, 1869–1939*. London: Routledge & Kegan Paul, 1985.

Rose, Nikolas, Rasmus Birk, and Nick Manning. "Towards Neuroecosociality: Mental Health in Adversity." *Theory, Culture & Society* 39, no. 3 (2022): 121–44. https://doi.org/10.1177/0263276420981614.

Rosenbaum, Susanna, and Ruti Talmor. "Self-Care." *Feminist Anthropology* 3, no. 2 (2022): 362–72. https://doi.org/10.1002/fea2.12088.

Russell, D. W. "UCLA Loneliness Scale (Version 3): Reliability, Validity, and Factor Structure." *Journal of Personality Assessment* 66, no. 1 (1996): 20–40. https://doi.org/10.1207/s15327752jpa6601_2.

Sauter, Theresa. "'What's on Your Mind?' Writing on Facebook as a Tool for Self-Formation." *New Media & Society* 16, no. 5 (2014): 823–39. https://doi.org/10.1177/1461444813495160.

Schaff, Kory P. "Foucault and the Critical Tradition." *Human Studies* 25, no. 3 (2002): 323–32.

Schneider, Christoph, Markus Weinmann, and Jan vom Brocke. "Digital Nudging: Guiding Online User Choices through Interface Design." *Communications of the ACM* 61, no. 7 (2018): 67–73. https://doi.org/10.1145/3213765.

Schultchen, Dana, Yannik Terhorst, Tanja Holderied, Michael Stach, Eva-Maria Messner, Harald Baumeister, and Lasse B. Sander. "Stay Present with Your Phone: A Systematic Review and Standardized Rating of Mindfulness Apps in European App Stores." *International Journal of Behavioral Medicine* 28, no. 5 (2021): 552–60. https://doi.org/10.1007/s12529-020-09944-y.

Schultz, Theodore W. "Investment in Human Capital." *American Economic Review* 51, no. 1 (1961): 1–17.

Seaver, Nick. "Captivating Algorithms: Recommender Systems as Traps." *Journal of Material Culture* 24, no. 4 (2019): 421–36. https://doi.org/10.1177/1359183518820366.

Sengers, Phoebe, Kirsten Boehner, Shay David, and Joseph "Jofish" Kaye. "Reflective Design." In *CC '05: Proceedings of the 4th Decennial Conference on Critical Computing: Between Sense and Sensibility*, 49–58.. New York: Association for Computing Machinery, 2005. https://doi.org/10.1145/1094562.1094569.

Shankar, Janki, Eugene Ip, Ernest Khalema, Jennifer Couture, Shawn Tan, Rosslynn T. Zulla, and Gavin Lam. "Education as a Social Determinant of Health: Issues Facing Indigenous and Visible Minority Students in Postsecondary Education in Western Canada." *International Journal of Environmental Research and Public Health* 10, no. 9 (2013): 3908–29. https://doi.org/10.3390/ijerph10093908.

Sibony, Anne-Lise. "The UK COVID-19 Response: A Behavioural Irony?" *European Journal of Risk Regulation* 11, no. 2 (2020): 350–57. https://doi .org/10.1017/err.2020.22.

Simon, Herbert Alexander. *Administrative Behavior: A Study of Decision-Making Processes in Administrative Organizations*. Fourth edition. New York: Free Press, 1997.

Smith, Daniel W. "Foucault on Ethics and Subjectivity: 'Care of the Self' and 'Aesthetics of Existence.'" *Foucault Studies*, no. 19 (June 2015): 135–50. https://doi.org/10.22439/fs.v0i19.4819.

———. "Two Concepts of Resistance:" In *Between Deleuze and Foucault*, edited by Daniel W. Smith, Nicolae Morar, and Thomas Nail, 264–82. Edinburgh: Edinburgh University Press, 2016.

Sointu, Eeva. "The Rise of an Ideal: Tracing Changing Discourses of Wellbeing." *The Sociological Review* 53, no. 2 (2005): 255–74. https://doi.org/10.1111 /j.1467-954X.2005.00513.x.

Spangler, Todd. "Facebook's Sheryl Sandberg: 'Not All Interactions in Social Media Are Equally Good for People.'" *Variety* (blog), February 28, 2018. https://variety.com/2018/digital/news/facebooks-sheryl-sandberg-social-media-well-being-1202713211/.

Specker Sullivan, Laura, and Peter Reiner. "Digital Wellness and Persuasive Technologies." *Philosophy & Technology* 34, no. 3 (2021): 413–24. https:// doi.org/10.1007/s13347-019-00376-5.

Spivak, Gayatri Chakravorty. *A Critique of Postcolonial Reason: Toward a History of the Vanishing Present*. Cambridge, MA: Harvard University Press, 1999.

Sridhar, Devi. "Social Media Could Be as Harmful to Children as Smoking or Gambling—Why Is This Allowed?" *The Guardian*, July 4, 2023. www .theguardian.com/commentisfree/2023/jul/04/smoking-gambling -children-social-media-apps-snapchat-health-regulation.

Stark, Luke. "Algorithmic Psychometrics and the Scalable Subject." *Social Studies of Science* 48, no. 2 (2018): 204–31. https://doi.org/10.1177 /0306312718772094.

Stearns, Peter N. *Shame: A Brief History*. Champaign: University of Illinois Press, 2017.

Steers, Mai-Ly N., Robert E. Wickham, and Linda K. Acitelli. "Seeing Everyone Else's Highlight Reels: How Facebook Usage Is Linked to Depressive Symptoms." *Journal of Social and Clinical Psychology* 33, no. 8 (2014): 701–31. https://doi.org/10.1521/jscp.2014.33.8.701.

Stypinska, Diana. *On the Genealogy of Critique: Or How We Have Become Decadently Indignant.* Abingdon, UK: Routledge, 2020.

———. *Social Media, Truth and the Care of the Self: On the Digital Technologies of the Subject.* Cham, Switzerland: Palgrave Macmillan, 2022.

Su, Norman Makoto, Amanda Lazar, and Lilly Irani. "Critical Affects: Tech Work Emotions amidst the Techlash." *Proceedings of the ACM on Human-Computer Interaction* 5, issue CSCW1 (April 2021): article 179. https://doi.org/10.1145/3449253.

Syvertsen, Trine, and Gunn Enli. "Digital Detox: Media Resistance and the Promise of Authenticity." *Convergence* 26, no. 5–6 (2020): 1269–83. https://doi.org/10.1177/1354856519847325.

Tandon, Anushree, Puneet Kaur, Amandeep Dhir, and Matti Mäntymäki. "Sleepless Due to Social Media? Investigating Problematic Sleep Due to Social Media and Social Media Sleep Hygiene." *Computers in Human Behavior* 113 (2020): 106487. https://doi.org/10.1016/j.chb.2020.106487.

Tao, Xiangyu, and Celia B. Fisher. "Exposure to Social Media Racial Discrimination and Mental Health among Adolescents of Color." *Journal of Youth and Adolescence* 51, no. 1 (2022): 30–44. https://doi.org/10.1007/s10964-021-01514-z.

Taylor, Charles. "Foucault on Freedom and Truth." *Political Theory* 12, no. 2 (1984): 152–83. https://doi.org/10.1177/0090591784012002002.

Terranova, Tiziana. "Attention, Economy and the Brain." *Culture Machine* 13 (2012).

Thaler, Richard H. *Misbehaving: The Making of Behavioral Economics.* New York: W. W. Norton, 2015.

Thaler, Richard H., and Cass R. Sunstein. *Nudge: Improving Decisions about Health, Wealth, and Happiness.* New Haven, CT: Yale University Press, 2008.

Thompson, Nicholas. "How Facebook Checks Facts and Polices Hate Speech." *Wired,* July 6, 2018. www.wired.com/story/how-facebook-checks-facts-and-polices-hate-speech/.

Tiidenberg, Katrin, Annette Markham, Gabriel Pereira, Mads Rehder, Ramona Dremljuga, Jannek K. Sommer, and Meghan Dougherty. "'I'm an Addict' and Other Sensemaking Devices: A Discourse Analysis of Self-Reflections on Lived Experience of Social Media." In *#SMSociety17: Proceedings of the 8th International Conference on Social Media & Society,* 1–10. New York: Association for Computing Machinery, 2017. https://doi.org/10.1145/3097286.3097307.

Tiisala, Tuomo. "Foucault, Neoliberalism, and Equality." *Critical Inquiry* 48, no. 1 (2021): 23–44. https://doi.org/10.1086/715986.

Tracy, Jessica L., and Richard W. Robins. "Putting the Self into Self-Conscious Emotions: A Theoretical Model." *Psychological Inquiry* 15, no. 2 (2004): 103–25. https://doi.org/10.1207/s15327965pli1502_01.

Traue, Boris. "The Cybernetic Self and Its Discontents: Care and Self-Care in the Information Society." In *Care or Control of the Self? Norbert Elias, Michel Foucault, and the Subject in the 21st Century*, edited by Andrea D. Bührmann and Stefanie Ernst, 158–78. Cambridge: Cambridge Scholars.

Trengove, Markus, Emre Kazim, Denise R. S. Almeida, Airlie Hilliard, Elizabeth Lomas, and Sara Zannone. "A Digital Duty of Care: A Critical Review of the Online Safety Bill." SSRN, April 1, 2022. https://doi.org/10.2139/ssrn.4072593.

Turland, James, Lynne Coventry, Debora Jeske, Pam Briggs, and Aad Van Moorsel. "Nudging towards Security: Developing an Application for Wireless Network Selection for Android Phones." In *British HCI '15: Proceedings of the 2015 British HCI Conference*, 193–201. New York: Association for Computing Machinery, 2015.

Valasek, Chad J. "Disciplining the Akratic User: Constructing Digital (Un)Wellness." *Mobile Media & Communication* 10, no. 2 (2022): 235–50. https://doi.org/10.1177/20501579211038796.

Valkenburg, Patti M. "Social Media Use and Well-Being: What We Know and What We Need to Know." *Current Opinion in Psychology* 45 (June 2022): 101294. https://doi.org/10.1016/j.copsyc.2021.12.006.

Valkenburg, Patti M., Irene I. van Driel, and Ine Beyens. "The Associations of Active and Passive Social Media Use with Well-Being: A Critical Scoping Review." *New Media & Society* 24, no. 2 (2022): 530–49.

Valverde, Mariana. *Diseases of the Will: Alcohol and the Dilemmas of Freedom.* Cambridge: Cambridge University Press, 1998.

van Wichelen, Sonja, and Marc de Leeuw. *Biolegality: A Critical Introduction.* Singapore: Springer Nature Singapore, 2024.

Vanden Abeele, Mariek M. P., Annabell Halfmann, and Edmund W. J. Lee. "Drug, Demon, or Donut? Theorizing the Relationship between Social Media Use, Digital Well-Being and Digital Disconnection." *Current Opinion in Psychology* 45 (June 2022): 101295. https://doi.org/10.1016/j.copsyc.2021.12.007.

Vandenbosch, Laura, Jasmine Fardouly, and Marika Tiggemann. "Social Media and Body Image: Recent Trends and Future Directions." *Current Opinion in Psychology* 45 (June 2022): 101289. https://doi.org/10.1016/j.copsyc.2021.12.002.

Verbeek, Peter-Paul. *Moralizing Technology: Understanding and Designing the Morality of Things*. Chicago: University of Chicago Press, 2011.

Verduyn, Philippe, Nino Gugushvili, and Ethan Kross. "Do Social Networking Sites Influence Well-Being? The Extended Active-Passive Model." *Current Directions in Psychological Science* 31, no. 1 (2022): 62–68. https://doi.org/10.1177/09637214211053637.

Verduyn, Philippe, Oscar Ybarra, Maxime Résibois, John Jonides, and Ethan Kross. "Do Social Network Sites Enhance or Undermine Subjective Well-Being? A Critical Review." *Social Issues and Policy Review* 11, no. 1 (2017): 274–302. https://doi.org/10.1111/sipr.12033.

Villa, Dana Richard. *Socratic Citizenship*. Princeton, NJ: Princeton University Press, 2001.

Wajcman, Judy. *Pressed for Time: The Acceleration of Life in Digital Capitalism*. Chicago: University of Chicago Press, 2016.

Walther, Joseph B. "Social Media and Online Hate." *Current Opinion in Psychology* 45 (June 2022): 101298. https://doi.org/10.1016/j.copsyc.2021.12.010.

Webb, Jennifer B., Erin R. Vinoski, Jan Warren-Findlow, Marlene I. Burrell, and Davina Y. Putz. "Downward Dog Becomes Fit Body, Inc.: A Content Analysis of 40 Years of Female Cover Images of *Yoga Journal*." *Body Image* 22 (September 2017): 129–35. https://doi.org/10.1016/j.bodyim.2017.07.001.

Weisgerber, Corinne, and Shannan H. Butler, "Curating the Soul: Foucault's Concept of *Hupomnemata* and the Digital Technology of Self-Care." *Information, Communication & Society* 19, no. 10 (2016): 1340–55.

Wells, Georgia, Jeff Horwitz, and Deepa Seetharaman. "Facebook Knows Instagram Is Toxic for Teen Girls, Company Documents Show." *The Wall Street Journal*, September 14, 2021. www.wsj.com/articles/facebook-knows-instagram-is-toxic-for-teen-girls-company-documents-show-11631620739.

Welsh, Talia. "The Affirmative Culture of Healthy Self-Care: A Feminist Critique of the Good Health Imperative." *IJFAB: International Journal of Feminist Approaches to Bioethics* 13, no. 1 (2020): 27–44. https://doi.org/10.3138/ijfab.13.1.02.

White, Richard. "Foucault on the Care of the Self as an Ethical Project and a Spiritual Goal." *Human Studies* 37, no. 4 (2014): 489–504. https://doi.org/10.1007/s10746-014-9331-3.

White, Sarah C. "Relational Wellbeing: Re-centring the Politics of Happiness, Policy and the Self." *Policy & Politics* 45, no. 2 (2017): 121–36.

Whitehead, Mark. "Neuroliberalism in the Digital Age: The Emerging Geographies of the Behavioural State." In *Handbook on the Changing Geographies of the State*, edited by Sami Moisio, Natalie Koch, Andrew E. G. Jonas, Christopher Lizotte, and Juho Luukkonen. Cheltenham, UK: Edward Elgar, 2020.

Whitehead, Mark, Rhys Jones, Rachel Lilley, Rachel Howell, and Jessica Pykett. "Neuroliberalism: Cognition, Context, and the Geographical Bounding of Rationality." *Progress in Human Geography* 43, no. 4 (2019): 632–49.

Whittle, Andrea, and André Spicer. "Is Actor Network Theory Critique?" *Organization Studies* 29, no. 4 (2008): 611–29. https://doi.org/10.1177/0170840607082223.

Wiener, Jonathan B. "The Regulation of Technology, and the Technology of Regulation." *Technology and Science Entering the 21st Century* 26, no. 2 (2004): 483–500. https://doi.org/10.1016/j.techsoc.2004.01.033.

Wilby, Peter. "By His Act of Betrayal, Clegg Will Lose His Greatest Reward." *The Guardian*, December 14, 2010. www.theguardian.com/commentisfree/2010/dec/14/betrayal-clegg-punish-alternative-vote.

Wilkinson, Richard G., and Michael Marmot. "Social Determinants of Health: The Solid Facts." Doc. no. EUR/ICP/CHVD 03 09 01, World Health Organization, Regional Office for Europe, 1998. https://apps.who.int/iris/handle/10665/108082.

Williams, Raymond. *Marxism and Literature*. Oxford: Oxford University Press, 1977.

Winner, Langdon. "Do Artifacts Have Politics?" *Daedalus* 109, no. 1 (1980): 121–36.

Wolfers, Lara N., and Sonja Utz. "Social Media Use, Stress, and Coping." *Current Opinion in Psychology* 45 (June 2022): 101305. https://doi.org/10.1016/j.copsyc.2022.101305.

Wolff, Robert Paul, Barrington Moore, and Herbert Marcuse. *A Critique of Pure Tolerance*. Boston: Beacon Press, 1969.

Wood, Joanne V. "What Is Social Comparison and How Should We Study It?" *Personality and Social Psychology Bulletin* 22, no. 5 (1996): 520–37. https://doi.org/10.1177/0146167296225009.

Woolgar, Steve. "Configuring the User: The Case of Usability Trials." *The Sociological Review* 38, no. 1 (1990): 58–99. https://doi.org/10.1111/j.1467-954X.1990.tb03349.x.

World Health Organization. "Social Determinants of Health." Accessed July 23, 2024. www.who.int/health-topics/social-determinants-of-health.

Yazdanipoor, Forouzan, Hady Faramarzi, and Abdollah Bicharanlou. "Digital Labour and the Generation of Surplus Value on Instagram." *tripleC: Communication, Capitalism & Critique* 20, no. 2 (2022): 179–94. https://doi.org/10.31269/triplec.v20i2.1304.

Yearby, Ruqaiijah. "Structural Racism and Health Disparities: Reconfiguring the Social Determinants of Health Framework to Include the Root Cause." *The Journal of Law, Medicine & Ethics* 48, no. 3 (2020): 518–26. https://doi.org/10.1177/1073110520958876.

Yoon, Sunkyung, Mary Kleinman, Jessica Mertz, and Michael Brannick. "Is Social Network Site Usage Related to Depression? A Meta-Analysis of Facebook–Depression Relations." *Journal of Affective Disorders* 248 (2019): 65–72. https://doi.org/10.1016/j.jad.2019.01.026.

Index

Page numbers followed by *n* refer to information in notes with the note number following the *n*. Multiple notes on the same page are denoted by *nn*.

Bergen, Jan Peter, 188

blame (idioms of user distress), 135, 137, 143, 145, 158. *See also* guilt and shame

bonding social capital, 64, 65, 66

bounded rationality, 92

Bourdieu, Pierre, 70, 72

bridging social capital, 64–65, 66

Briggs, Charles, 120, 124

British Facebook users. *See* Facebook users (qualitative interview study)

Brock, André L., 209n135

Brown, Wendy, 74, 97

Bucher, Taina, 36, 88, 107, 132, 225n22

Burke, Moira, 52, 53, 54–55, 60, 109

Butler, Judith, 47, 169, 170

Cadman, Louisa, 169, 204n97

Cambridge Analytica case, 44, 47, 211n24

Canguilhem, Georges, 42–43, 168

capitalism: co-optation, 183; counter-conduct (and care of the self) tactics, 179, 183; Facebook's design, 55–56, 76, 77–78, 89, 112; and Facebook's healthy user configuration, 37, 43–44, 57–59, 63, 78; neoliberal governmentalities, 27; social media tools of well-being, 83; through datafication, 4, 5, 18, 55–56, 89, 112; user well-being/ individual habits correlation, 5, 9; well-being, capitalist capacity for, 179, 231n62; wellness influencer posts, 156

care of the self, 29, 39, 176, 190; hermeneutic of mediation, 188–89; power in the Hellenistic world, 173, 183; self-care as warfare/resistance, 180–81; self-relation, 172–73, 175, 179–80, 183–84, 190; and the

sociotechnical view, 185–89. *See also* self-care

Center for Humane Technology, 24, 203–4n89

choice architects. *See* nudge

Chun, Wendy, 33

class and social capital, 70–71

Clegg, Nick, 81, 217–18n8

Coleman, James S., 68–69

coloniality of power, 62

comments (on posts): active/passive binary, 52–53; as bonding social capital, 65; datafication, 56; design of, 111; and Facebook ranking, 109, 223n80; kindness reminders, 82–83; mediation, 187

communities: Facebook's evolutionary discourse, 110; hate as a prosocial phenomenon, 14; in the limit attitude, 169, 170; living well, models of, 75, 180, 183, 196n30; peer support, 16; and responsibilization, 8

comparison, social. *See* social comparison

congealed labor, 103, 104

connected obligation, 146–50

co-optation, 183

corporate responsibility, 52, 83–84

counter-conduct, 29, 39, 171–72, 176–79, 230n33

COVID-19 pandemic, 25–26, 95, 119, 134–35

Cox, Chris, 50–51

Cramer, Florian, 104

critical medical humanities, 22

critical researchers, 37, 59, 114, 161. *See also* refusal (of the neoliberal terms of well-being)

critical technocultural discourse analysis (CTDA), 209n135

curation (user curation of Facebook Feed), 107–8, 142–44

dark patterns (of social media design), 8, 24, 86
datafication, 4, 5; attention-grabbing fury, 18; dark patterns, tactics of, 24; Facebook's design, 55–56, 77–78, 89, 112; and Facebook's healthy user configuration, 43–44, 57–59, 63, 78, 114; metrification (likes and emojis), 212n28; new reflections of healthy use, 179; social media tools of well-being, 83; well-being apps, 84. *See also* attention economy
Davidson, Arnold, 171
Davies, William, 67
defaults in design, 90–91, 101–2, 109
depression: and the ambivalent force of social media, 160; contextual structural determinants, 22, 73, 75, 77; and Facebook's psycho-computational configuration of healthy use, 78; idioms of distress (expressed by Facebook users), 142, 158; and individual self-control, 20; and passive social media use, 2, 75; smartphones and rising mental health issues (teens, US), 15; social comparison (Facebook), 14
design: apparatuses of governance, 3, 6, 8–9; dark patterns, 8, 24, 86; defaults, 90–91, 101–2, 109; Facebook's monetization of natural needs, 55, 57, 58–59, 77–78; liberal paternalism, 38, 93–94, 118, 144; nudge, 81–82, 85, 86, 90–91, 93–94; and processes of inscription, 35, 36, 45–46; in the psycho-computational complex, 37, 48; rhetorical

operation of, 85–86, 100–103; to extract value, 24, 55–56, 76, 77–78, 84, 89, 112; and the tool-view of technology, 85; well-being apps, 84. *See also* design (of Facebook's Feed)
designed distrust, 38, 113, 117–18, 163
designed sociality, 56–57
design (of Facebook's Feed), 38, 86–87, 89; for active use, 51; datafication, 55–56, 77–78, 89, 112; defaults, 90–91, 109, 114; HCI research's justification, 63–64, 109; monetizing natural needs, 55, 57, 58–59, 77–78; neoliberal inequalities, 78; neuroliberal governance, 105; *News Feed FYI* blogs, 109; nudge, 38, 96, 105, 107–13, 114, 115–16, 163
Deville, Joe, 131
Dewey, John, 1, 33–34
digital detox, 24, 203n88
digital labor, 56
disciplinary power, 207n116. *See also* visibility, disciplinary regime of
discourses (of social media use and well-being): as apparatuses of governance, 3, 6, 8–9, 47; processes of inscription, 35, 36, 45–46. *See also* Facebook's discourses of user well-being
distress, idioms of. *See* idioms of distress (guilt and shame)
distrust, designed, 38, 113, 117–18, 163
Dolata, Ulrich, 150
Dorrestijn, Steven, 188–89

Egebark, Johan, 101
Ekström, Mathias, 101
Elmer, Greg, 78

employment: access to social capital, 64–65, 70–71; self-employment and connected obligation, 149–50; unemployment as a source of shame, 131, 158–59, 160

Enli, Gunn, 19

ethics: active/passive binary, 185; Buddhist traditions of detachment, 182; care of the self and self-care, 173, 179–83; and the limit attitude, 166, 168, 170; of neuroliberalism, 97–99; nudges, 85, 93–96, 112, 114, 116; positive computing, 84, 102; sociotechnical view of technology, 76, 187–89. *See also* topical exclusion

Eurocentricism, 121, 200n63

evolutionary biology, and Facebook's notifications, 139

evolutionary narratives of human belonging, 13, 37, 162–63; core argument of, 54–55; and Facebook's global expansion, 61–62; in a grid of intelligibility, 163; monetization of natural needs, 55, 57, 58–59, 77–78; and nudge, 96, 113, 117–18; relational investment, 60, 66

"Facebook Files" series (*Wall Street Journal*), 18

Facebook's discourses of user well-being, 36–37, 96, 162–63; active/passive use binary, 50–51, 52–53, 54; and alternative transparencies, 113, 114, 115; analytical approach to, 9, 44, 53–54; datafication, 43–44, 57–59, 63, 78, 114; *Hard Questions* (blog series), 51–53, 61, 62; neoliberalism, 67, 68, 69, 70–74, 75, 77, 78, 113; *News Feed FYI* (Facebook blog), 108–9, 111; social

capital, 60–61, 64–73, 78; Zuckerberg's US Senate Committee testimony, 44, 46–47, 48, 49–50. *See also* evolutionary narratives of human belonging

Facebook's Feed: history of, 87, 106; neuroliberal governance, 89, 104–5, 112, 113, 114, 116; political critiques and controversies, 87–88; ranking, 87, 88, 108–10, 112, 222–23n80; visibility, disciplinary regime of, 88–89, 107, 130. *See also* design (of Facebook's Feed); Facebook users (qualitative interview study)

Facebook users (qualitative interview study), 38–39; connected obligation, 146–50; interview procedure, 119–21, 123–25; self-nudge, 122, 138–46, 147, 150, 153; well-being, user understandings of, 150–53. *See also* idioms of distress (guilt and shame)

Fast, Karin, 19

fault. *See* blame (idioms of user distress)

feeling. *See* structures of feeling

Ferragina, Emanuele, 69

financial crash (2008 and global recession), 97–98

Fisher, Matthew, 73

Foot, Philippa, 57

Forlizzi, Jodi, 101–2

Foucault, Michel: apparatuses of power, 3, 31–32, 43, 45, 206n113, 207n116; axes of analysis (knowledge, power, ethics), 162–64, 166; care of the self, 172, 173, 180, 184; counter-conduct, 230n33; and governance, 3, 27–28, 49, 163; habits, 1, 207n116; limit attitude, 166–70; and neoliberalism, 27, 67,

69–70, 180; panoptic discipline, 88;
parrēsia, 174–75; subjectivation, 28,
163, 212n27
Fraser, Nancy, 160
free subjects, 167, 171, 173
Friedman, Milton, 94
Fuchs, Christian, 56
Fuller, Matthew, 35, 104

Galen, 42
gambling industry, 98, 221n54
gender, 17, 132, 210–11n17
Gershon, Ilana, 88
Gigerenzer, Gerd, 99, 100
Gillespie, Tarleton, 79
Ginsberg, David, 52
Goffey, Andrew, 35
Golder, Ben, 9, 171
governance, 3, 27–29, 49, 170–71. *See
also* neuroliberal governance
governments: care of the self,
importance of, 183–84; coalition
government (UK, 2010), 217–18n8;
nudge policies, 25–26, 94–95; public
health policies, 19–20, 25–26, 74, 95,
98, 136–37, 221n54; US Senate
(Zuckerberg's 2018 testimony to),
44, 46–47, 48, 49–50. *See also*
liberal democracy
Gramsci, Antonio, 161, 226n32
Granovetter, Mark, 64
Grosser, Benjamin, 88
Guggenheim, Michael, 131
guilt and shame: addiction and
technological guilt, 136, 137; and
apparatuses of power, 39, 122–23,
135, 145, 158, 160; from normative
comparison, 130, 131, 132, 158–59;
functions of, 153–58; responsibilization, costs of, 123, 158–61, 164
Guthman, Julie, 136–37

Haidt, Jonathan, 15
Hall, Stuart, 40
Hard Questions (Facebook blog
series), 51–53, 61, 62
Hassard, John, 208n130
hate, 14, 127
Haugen, Frances, 50
HCI research. *See* human-computer
interaction (HCI) research (funded
by Facebook)
health (general): exposome, 22;
historico-cultural frameworks,
41–42; nudge tactics, 82, 102;
personal habits, contemporary
focus on, 2; public health policies,
19–20, 25–26, 74, 95, 98, 136–37,
221n54; relational norms, 42–43;
well-being apps, 84–85, 94. *See also*
social determinants of health
"Healthy Social Media Habits: How
You Use It Matters" (National
Institutes of Health), 19–20
herd mentality, 91–92
historico-critical attitude. *See* limit
attitude
Hookway, Branden, 103
Hrdličková, Zuzana, 131
human-computer interaction (HCI)
research (funded by Facebook), 37,
53; and the active/passive binary,
50–51, 52–53, 54, 65–66, 68; design
(of Facebook's Feed), 63–64, 109,
114; evolutionary discourses, 54–55,
57, 61; proprietorial enframing, 52,
78; and the psycho-computational
complex, 44, 48, 49, 52, 64; relationship maintenance and investment,
60, 66; social capital, 64–65, 68–69

idioms of distress (guilt and shame):
addiction, 117, 135–37, 149;

power (continued)
    self), 29, 171, 175, 177, 181, 183–84,
    189; digital distress, individualized
    experiences of, 39, 122–23, 135, 145,
    158, 160, 164; disciplinary regime
    of visibility, 88–89, 107, 130;
    Foucault's axis of power, 162, 163;
    Foucault's *dispositif,* 31–32, 207n116;
    juridico-discursive matrix, 30–31;
    micropolitics of nudge (in
    Facebook's Feed), 104, 114;
    relational views of health and
    well-being, 22; through technologi-
    cal scripts, 35, 37, 43; topical
    exclusion, 23, 72. *See also* govern-
    ance; neuroliberal governance
privacy settings, 107
proprietorial enframing, 52, 78
psycho-computational complex,
    45–49, 74, 170. *See also* psycho-
    computational complex (Facebook)
psycho-computational complex
    (Facebook), 37, 44, 54; Feed as
    neuroliberal interface, 105;
    governance, 49, 78; *Hard Questions*
    blog series, 52; HCI research, 44, 48,
    49, 52, 64; idioms of (user) distress,
    155; and structural inequalities, 78;
    Zuckerberg's US Senate Committee
    testimony, 44, 46–47, 48, 49–50
psy-disciplines, 11–18, 21, 96. *See also*
    human-computer interaction (HCI)
    research (funded by Facebook)
public health policies, 19–20, 25–26,
    74, 95, 98, 136–37, 221n54

"quiet" modes. *See* notification
    management
Quijano, Aníbal, 62
quitting social media, 176. *See also*
    connected obligation

Rabinow, Paul, 165
Rajchman, John, 184
ranking (Facebook Feed), 87, 88,
    108–10, 112, 222–23n80
rational limits (of humans), 90–93, 95,
    100, 103, 113, 163
Rebonato, Riccardo, 93
Redström, Johan, 85, 86
refusal (of the neoliberal terms of
    well-being), 39, 59, 63, 77–80,
    165–66, 171. *See also* care of the self;
    counter-conduct; limit attitude
relational approaches to well-being,
    73–76. *See also* social determinants
    of health
relational habits, 33–35, 36
relational investment, 60, 66
relationship maintenance, 60, 62, 65,
    110
resistances, 29, 116. *See also* care of the
    self; counter-conduct; limit
    attitude; refusal (of the neoliberal
    terms of well-being)
responsibilization, 185, 189; and
    critics of social media, 8, 23–24,
    29–30; defined, 8, 123, 195n22;
    idioms of distress (expressed by
    Facebook users), 39, 123, 143,
    158–61, 164; neoliberal health (non)
    intervention, 19–20, 25, 74, 136–37,
    182, 201–2n71; new reflections on
    healthy use, 177, 178; operationali-
    zation through self-nudge (by
    Facebook users), 138, 145, 153;
    public campaigns for present-day
    issues, 98; and the tool-view of
    technology, 30. *See also* neuroliberal
    governance
Rommes, Else, 45
Rose, Nikolas, 11–12, 26, 43, 49,
    197n35

Founded in 1893,
UNIVERSITY OF CALIFORNIA PRESS
publishes bold, progressive books and journals
on topics in the arts, humanities, social sciences,
and natural sciences—with a focus on social
justice issues—that inspire thought and action
among readers worldwide.

The UC PRESS FOUNDATION
raises funds to uphold the press's vital role
as an independent, nonprofit publisher, and
receives philanthropic support from a wide
range of individuals and institutions—and from
committed readers like you. To learn more, visit
ucpress.edu/supportus.